A. Neiger

Atlas
of Practical Proctology

Compliments of KARL STORZ

A. Neiger

Atlas of Practical Proctology

Second completely revised and expanded edition
Translated from the German by Thomas A. Crozier

Foreword by John Alexander-Williams

Hogrefe & Huber Publishers
Toronto • Lewiston, NY • Bern • Göttingen • Stuttgart

Library of Congress Cataloging-in-Publication Data

Neiger, A.
    [Atlas der praktischen Proktologie. English]
    Atlas of practical proctology / A. Neiger. — 2nd completely rev. and expanded ed.
    p. cm.
    Translation of: Atlas der praktischen Proktologie.
1. Proctology—Atlases. I. Title.
[DNLM: 1. Colon—surgery—atlases. 2. Rectum—surgery—atlases. WI 17 N397a]
RC864.N3613   1990   616.3'5—dc20   89-71714 CIP

Canadian Cataloguing in Publication Data

Neiger, A.
    Atlas of practical proctology

2nd completely rev. and expanded ed.
Includes bibliographical references.

RC864.N44   1990   616.3'5   C90-093261-9

P. O. Box 51
Lewiston, NY 14092

12–14 Bruce Park Ave.
Toronto, Ontario M4P 2S3

ISBN 0-920887-76-7
ISBN 3-456-81879-3
Hogrefe & Huber Publishers • Toronto • Lewiston, NY • Bern • Göttingen • Stuttgart

Printed by E. Schoop AG, Urnäsch, Switzerland
Photos and lithography: Henzi AG, Bern, Switzerland
Printed in Switzerland

Table of Contents

Foreword

Dr. Neiger, in the Preface to the 1st Edition, refers to proctology as a "cinderella" specialty. This perception, true some years ago, is changing. It is changing largely because of the calibre of the men and women in the field. It is changing because proctological specialists are becoming more innovative, scientific and communicative. Dr. Neiger is one of those who has done much to improve the image of proctology because he is a practical proctologist and a skillful communicator. He has long experience as a specialist, a keen eye as an observer, and a logical mind that organises the most efficient and practical steps in achieving the correct diagnosis and the best treatment.

At one time it was reasonable to describe proctology as a specialty falling between two stools or maybe among four specialties. To use another metaphor, proctology used to have one foot in the camp of surgery, another in dermatology, and perhaps its arms in venerology and internal medicine. It could be described as being spread-eagled with its eye firmly fixed on the fundament! This image is now changing rapidly. Proctology has become an integral part of hind-gut surgery, which ranges from pouches to piles. It has become a "macho" subspecialty, requiring high technical surgical skills in the creation of pouches, in the restoration of continence and the preservation of the anal sphincter in rectal cancer surgery. The management of anal ills nestles at the quieter, gentler end of the specialty. However, it has not been neglected in the march of progress, and we have proctologists like Dr. Alex Neiger to thank for that.

For me the striking feature of this book is the high quality of the photography and the clarity of the accompanying line drawings. Another bonus for English-speaking readers is the extensive bibliography, with references to many articles written in German and French. This should widen the knowledge and perspective of the English-speaking specialists.

Although designed primarily as a book for general practitioners, it will be read by candidates for surgical examinations and, in one of its many translations, must be on the book shelves of all self-respecting proctologist and colorectal surgeon around the world.

In other corners of the world, there are proctologists who prefer slight variations to the techniques of diagnosis and therapy shown in this book. Some have the facilities to tip their patients anus-upwards on expensive, electrically motored couches and, perhaps, even more who examine their patients in the left lateral position, despite the wear and tear on their own cervical spines. There are some specialists who are sceptical about cryptitis as a pathological entity, and those who adopt slightly different regimens for the application of photocoagulation. However much we may be at minor variance with some of the necessarily didactic points in this practical manual, his fellow specialists are united in one thing—admiration for this magnificent achievement and our envy at his exceptional collection of slides. The enthusiastic reception of this book is a just reward to Dr. Neiger for all the painstaking acquisition of teaching material and the many hours spent preparing the work.

J. Alexander-Williams, MD, FRCS
Professor of Gastrointestinal Surgery,
Birmingham, UK

Preface

Dr. Neiger having kindly invited me to contribute a preface to the present work, I am happy to take this opportunity to pay tribute to his tireless activity in the proctological field. Imbued with a rare enthusiasm for this branch of medicine and endowed with great technical skill, coupled with a remarkable clinical flair, he is now widely acknowledged as a proctologist of authority. After spending a few years as an assistant in my clinic, he set up practice as a specialist in Bern, where he also continues to act as head of the outpatient department for proctology at the University Outpatient Clinic. His various sojourns abroad have likewise served to broaden both his theoretical and particularly his practical knowledge. Thanks to his keen interest and manual dexterity we have been able to make such extensive and profitable use of the latest developments in endoscopy. His new atlas, incidentally, also testifies to his talents as a photographer.

The chief value of endoscopy lies in the wealth of information it provides, while at the same time imposing relatively little strain on the patient. Since endoscopic examinations can, in most cases, be carried out on an ambulant basis, there is great scope for them in out-patient departments and in domestic practice. At a time when hospital costs are rising by leaps and bounds, and nursing staff is in such short supply, it is of major advantage to be able to undertake diagnostic procedures in the consulting room. Hence, the importance of the present book, which is designed to familiarise the practicing physician with a medical discipline about which most doctors known far too little. It would be wrong, moreover, to regard this work merely as an atlas. The brief and simple text accompanying the illustrations makes the book a genuine proctological compendium, which should undoubtedly achieve all that its author intended.

Prof. F. Reubi
Director of the University
Medical Outpatient Clinic, Bern

Preface to the First Edition

It all began with a number of slides that I had taken over the years in my proctological practice and in the outpatient department of the University Clinic for Internal Medicine in Bern, Switzerland. Since these pictures afford a good survey of proctological diseases, I wanted to make them available to a larger audience.

I felt that proctology had been treated like medicine's poor relation; there were not enough well-trained proctologists. I knew that there were a large number of patients with proctological complaints who had to depend on a relatively small number of colleagues who had the necessary training in the skills of proctology.

Most patients with proctological complaints consult their general practitioner, who may have had little or no formal training in proctology. So it was the general practitioner that I had in mind when I decided to produce this illustrated book. Since the general practitioner's time is limited, I decided to make this essentially a practical illustrated guide to proctology with a minimum of text. I tried to distill the essence of specialist proctological practice into an illustrated guide for the general practitioner. Therefore, exhaustive accounts of the treatment of all obscure diseases and complicated procedures seemed inappropriate. Readers stimulated to know more are referred to specialist literature. I have tried to concentrate on describing easily understood diagnostic and therapeutic procedures, and to accompany them with pictures and, where necessary, drawings of the techniques and instruments. I have deliberately excluded more complicated procedures such as flexible sigmoidoscopy and coloscopy, as these are usually employed only by specialists.

Inevitably, the practice of proctology overlaps with that of general surgery, internal medi-

cine, and dermatology, which is why the general practitioner is the ideal target for this book. It is particularly important that the general practitioner bear this in mind and not miss the diagnosis of venereal infections of the anal region, so a separate chapter on them has been included.

The publication of this *Atlas of Practical Proctology* in the present, profusely illustrated form would not have been possible without the generous support of the CIBA-GEIGY AG. I am indebted to their department for medical and pharmaceutical information, especially to Dr. H. Kaiser for editorial assistance and to Mr. J. Emmenegger for technical supervision. I owe thanks to Prof. H. Fahrländer, gastroenterologist in Basel, Switzerland, for his valuable suggestions. For donating valuable illustrations I am grateful to Dr. G. Clémencon, gastroenterologist in Olten; Prof. L. Eckmann, Director of the University Hospital, Tiefenausspital in Bern, Switzerland; Prof. W. Mohr, Director of the Bernhard Nocht Institute for Tropical Diseases in Hamburg; Dr. P. Otto, Department of Internal Medicine, Medical School in Hanover; Dr. M. Parturier-Albot, specialist for proctology in Paris; Prof. H. Stirnemann, Surgical Department of the District Hospital in Burgdorf, Switzerland; and Prof. A. Welchert, Surgical Clinic of the University of Lund in Malmö, Sweden.

The intentions of this book will have been fulfilled if I succeed in awakening increased interest for proctology in my colleagues in general practice, and if I help them to conduct a thorough proctological examination, leading to a correct diagnosis and appropriate treatment.

Dr. med. A. Neiger

Preface to the Third German Edition

The great interest shown toward the previous two German editions and those in French, English, Spanish and Portuguese, proved that there is a demand for didactic aids in the form of short, illustrated texts describing the diagnosis and treatment of proctological disorders. A new edition has become necessary to do justice to new discoveries. Thanks to the generosity of the companies of Dr. Falk in Freiburg i.Br., West Germany, and Phardi AG in Basel, Switzerland, not only was a new edition, but also a considerable extension of both text and illustrations made possible. Additional chapters were added dealing with the anatomy of the rectum, the signs and symptoms of proctological diseases, and the most common findings seen on inspection. There are new chapters on the conservative therapy of hemorrhoids, anal pruritus, and ischemic colitis. The number of illustrations was almost doubled. This was possible since lithographs were available from numerous publications in various journals such as the *Schweiz. Medizinische Rundschau (PRAXIS)* published by Hallwag in Bern, *Hexagon Roche* published by Hoffmann-La Roche & Co. in Basel, *Colo-Proctology* published by Edition Nymphenburg in Munich, the *internistische praxis* published by Hans Marseille in Munich, as well as the journal *Musik und Medizin* of the I.M.P. Publishing Company in Neu-Isenberg.

I owe special thanks to Prof. Dr. med. A. Akovbiantz, Director of the Surgical Clinic of the Waldspital in Zurich; Dr. med. M. Flepp, Department for Infectious Diseases of the Outpatient Clinic for Internal Medicine in Zurich; Prof. Dr. med. P. Kiefhaber, Director of the Department for Internal Medicine of the Municipal Hospital in Traunstein; Dr. med. I. Lentini, Centro Proctologico in Barcelona; Dr. R. Münch, University Hospital in Zurich; Dr. med. E. Parnaud, Département de Proctologie, Hôpital des Diaconesses in Paris; and Prof. Dr. med. T. Rufli, Dermatological Clinic of the University of Basel for donating important illustrations. Prof. Dr. med. F. Gloor from the Institute of Pathology of the Canton Hospital in St. Gallen kindly gave me advice concerning inflammatory bowel diseases. I was advised by Dr. med. J.-O. Gebbers from the Institute of Pathology of the Canton Hospital of Lucerne about neoplasias, by Prof. Dr. med. K. Gyr, Head of Internal Medicine at the Canton Hospital in Liestal about amebiasis, and by Dr. med. H. Kaiser, specialist for dermatology in Freiburg i.Br. about sexually transmitted anorectal diseases. To keep printing costs down, I omitted photomicrographs.

We hope that with the help of the numerous illustrations and the brief text the reader will be able to find the necessary information quickly, even during consulting hours.

Dr. med. A. Neiger

Acknowledgement

The author wishes to thank Professor J. Alexander-Williams for the revision of the text and his many helpful suggestions.

Approach to the Patient with Anorectal Disorders

In proctology, as in all fields of medicine, it is essential to take an accurate history. This can provide information about possible familial disposition to disease such as varicose veins, hemorrhoids, cancer, or polyposis, while a precise description of the complaints with regard to onset (acute versus gradual), duration, symptom-free intervals, etc., greatly aids the diagnosis. This information is best gathered by direct questioning, since patients tend to forget important details in the unpleasant setting of their first proctological consultation. Sympathetic questioning helps the patient to overcome inhibitions and leads to an atmosphere of trust and understanding, which is particularly of importance in the diagnosis of sexually transmitted anorectal diseases. As the incidence of such diseases has increased greatly in recent years, this etiology must always be kept in mind.

Characteristic signs and symptoms of anorectal diseases are itching, pain, burning sensations, anal discharge (bloody, purulent, or mucoid), and difficulties in defecation. It is important to define the quality of the pain (stabbing, cutting, throbbing, dull) and its temporal relationship to defecation, as well as to determine the presence and nature of anorectal bleeding (dripping, spurting, mixed with the stool or simply layered on it). The combination of symptoms and their individual characteristics allow a presumptive diagnosis to be made, which is then often confirmed by the proctological examination.

In the following chapters, the symptoms are first listed in the order of their relative frequency. They are then described in detail in the context of specific diseases.

Signs and Symptoms of Anorectal Diseases

Bleeding and pain are the most common symptoms, followed in importance by anal discharge, itching, sensation of a foreign body in the rectum, a feeling of incomplete defecation with constant defecation urge (tenesmus), and changes in the character of the stool.

Bleeding

Traces of blood on the toilet paper are seen with eczema, fissure-in-ano, prolapsed mucosa or hemorrhoids, anal tumors, and also rarely in colitis ulcerative. Spurts of blood are seen with internal hemorrhoids. The passage of blood together with the stool is observed with colitis or rectum tumors. Blood is found layered on the stool with internal hemorrhoids, and with anal or rectum tumors [156].

Pain

Acute or gradually developing pain with a feeling of tension is experienced with thrombosed external hemorrhoids and abscesses. The pain of anal fissure is sharp and cutting, while anal abscess or cryptitis causes a dull aching in the anal canal.

Anal Discharge

The secretions of internal prolapse or solitary ulcer are clear, while those of proctitis are a yellowish brown. The discharge is purulent with colitis and fistulas, and watery or slightly tinged with blood in prolapse of the mucosa or rectum.

Pruritus

Pruritus is found with dermatitis or rarely with tumors in the anal region. Oxyuriasis (pinworms) causes nocturnal itching.

Defecation Urge

Space-occupying lesions such as prolapsed hemorrhoids, mucosa prolapse, rectal procidentia, or tumors cause a feeling of a foreign body in the anus and the urge to try to pass it.

Defecation Problems

Frequent passage of solid or pasty stools is a symptom or ulcerative colitis or tumors of the rectum or sigmoid colon. Constipation is a symptom of Hirschsprung's disease, and diverticulosis or stenosis of the sigmoid colon.

Anatomy of the Anus and Rectum

The distal boundary of the anal canal is formed by perianal skin covered by a deeply pigmented, stratified squamous epithelium that is hairless except for the anal verge. This skin merges proximally into the radially folded, grayish-blue, dull anoderm, which is covered by an only slightly cornified squamous epithelium extending to the pectinate line. A venous plexus—the inferior venous plexus, also known as the external hemorrhoidal plexus—lies under the distal anoderm. When the patient strains, this plexus can appear as an engorged ring and may be mistaken for prolapsing internal hemorrhoids. Thromboses in this plexus appear acutely as painful masses known as acute thrombotic hemorrhoids, external anal thrombosis, or thrombosed external hemorrhoids.

An approximately 0.7–2 cm wide transition zone covered with a variable stratified cuboid or columnar epithelium begins proximal to the pectinate line. Five to ten longitudinal folds of the mucous membrane called anal columns (Columnae rectales, columns of Morgagni) are found here. Between these lie the anal sinuses, which terminate in the anal crypts into which the anal glands empty. The latter were first described by Albrecht von Haller in 1751 [91]. The distal ends of the anal columns in the region of the pectinate line can be thickened and are then referred to as anal papillae. These may be mistaken for internal hemorrhoids if they are inflamed and swollen. The corpus cavernosum recti (internal hemorrhoidal plexus) lies just proximal to the pectinate line. This is an arteriovenous erectile tissue (cavernous tissue) situated under the epithelial transition zone [251, 252] which is supplied by the superior rectal artery. Venous blood drains through the anal sphincter into the rectal veins and into the inferior vena cava. Obstructions to venous drainage (especially with raised anal sphincter tone) and/or an increased arterial inflow lead to dilations of the thin-walled vessels of the arteriovenous plexus, which can tear during defecation and give rise to bright red bleeding. The rectal mucosa, a pale-pink, shiny, mobile simple cylindrical epithelium with prominent vascularization, begins proximal to the transition zone [13, 77, 182, 234, 251, 252, 262, 263, 264].

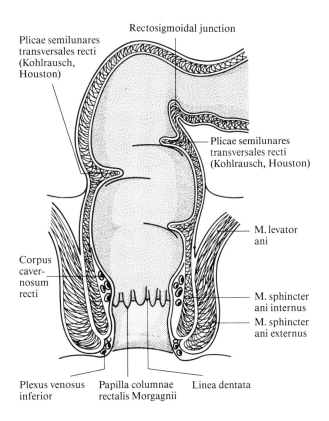

FIGURE 1
Anatomy of the anus and rectum.

Proctological Examination

History

The first proctological examinations were performed 4500 B.C. in ancient Egypt. Illustrations in the library of Leyden dating from the 14th century show that palpation of the rectum was known in the Middle Ages. The first rectoscope—in fact a universal endoscope with candle light—was used in Vienna in 1810 by Bozzini [117]. In 1853, the Parisian surgeon Désormeaux developed another rectoscope, which was a thin metal tube illuminated by a spirit lamp [9]. Larger-bored instruments were introduced around the turn of the century. The rigid tube design with illumination (now provided from a cold-light source via fiber-glass bundles) has proved to be useful to the present day. Flexible fiberoptic instruments have extended the range of endoscopy to sigmoidoscopic and coloscopic examinations [48, 116, 124, 156, 280].

Modern Examination

Today, a full proctological examination should be performed whenever the patient has one or more of the following:

– pain in the anorectal region,

– bloody or mucoid discharge from the anus,

– changes in bowel habit.

A rectoscopic examination should also be performed as part of every radiological examination of the colon, since fine changes in the rectum such as minute (pinhead-sized) polyps, early infiltrative processes, or proctitis can only be diagnosed by endoscopy.

A proctological examination including inspection of the anal region, palpation, and anoscopy should precede every endoscopic evaluation of more proximal portions of the colon (sigmoidoscopy, coloscopy), since diseases of the anorectal region are apt to be overlooked.

The steps of a complete proctological examination are

– inspection of the perianal region,

– digital examination,

– endoscopy.

Inspection of the Perianal Region

The best position for inspecting the perianal region is with the patient in the knee-elbow position and the buttocks spread widely. This position is better than when the patient lies on the side or back, as one can easily view the entire anal region. As well, in this position proctoscopy and rectoscopy can easily be carried out. Good lighting is essential. Anal eczema, rhagades, condylomas, external orifices of fistula, perianal thrombosis, skin protuberances (piles, sentinel tags), prolapsed hemorrhoids and polyps, abscesses, prolapse of the rectum, and malignancies can be detected. Straining as at defecation engorges external hemorrhoids and makes them visible, while internal hemorrhoids tend to prolapse. However, it is often necessary to perform the inspection immediately after defecation, since prolapse sometimes only occurs then.

The examination of the inguinal region for enlarged or painful lymph nodes is essential for the diagnosis of sexually transmitted diseases.

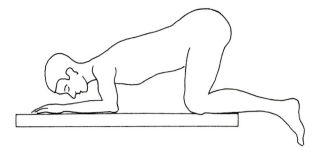

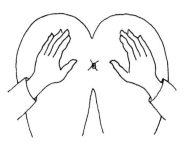

FIGURE 2
With the patient in the knee-elbow or knee-chest position the buttocks are gently spread and the anus is inspected (see Figure 5).

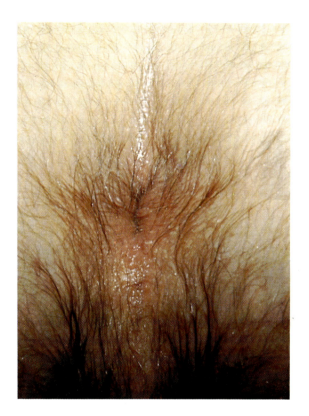

FIGURE 3
Normal anus.

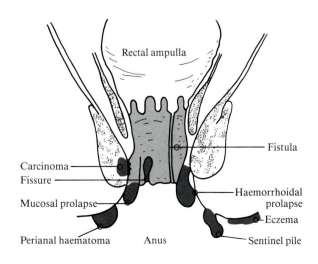

FIGURE 4
Diagram of anal diseases.

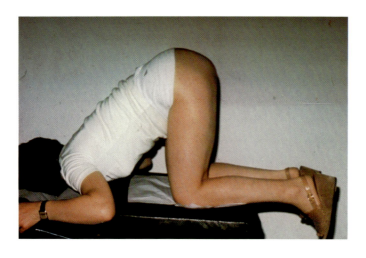

FIGURE 5
Knee-chest position on normal examina-
tion table.

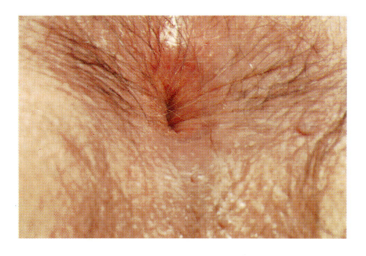

FIGURE 6
Inspection of normal anoderm. The anus
can be seen after the buttocks have been
spread.

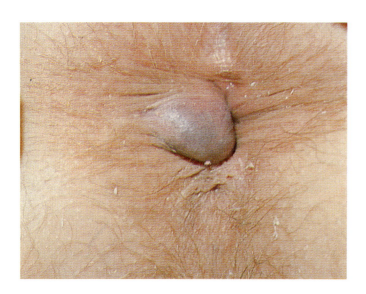

FIGURE 7
Thrombosed external hemorrhoid (peri-
anal thrombosis).

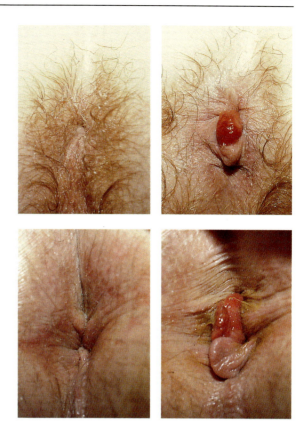

FIGURE 8
Pile prolapse during straining.

FIGURE 9
Partial mucosal prolapse during straining.

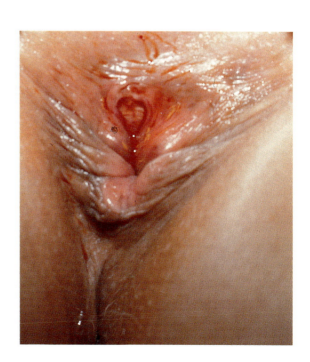

FIGURE 10
Fissure-in-ano.

18

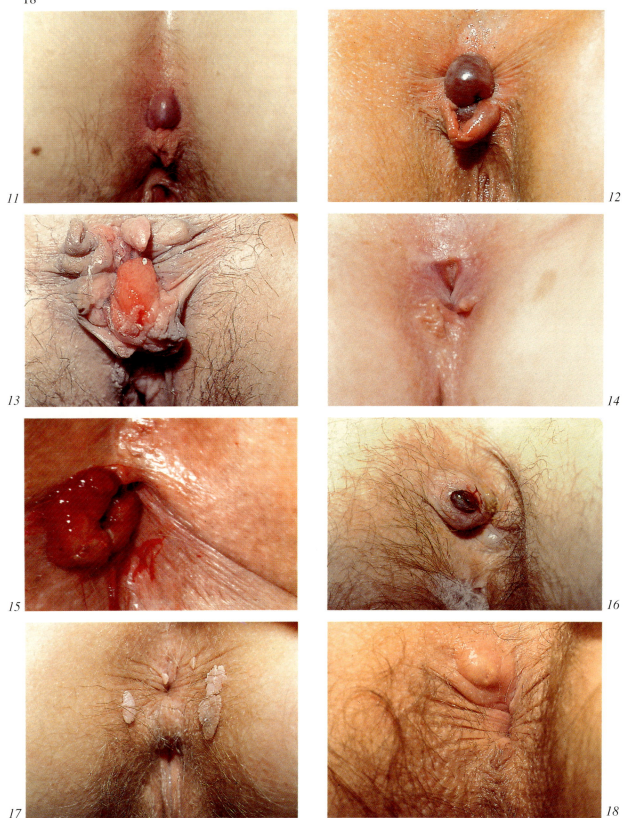

FIGURES 11–18
From left to right: perianal thrombosis, prolapsed pile, partial mucosal prolapse, fissure-in-ano, anal carcinoma, ulcerated perianal thrombosis, condyloma accuminata, abscess.

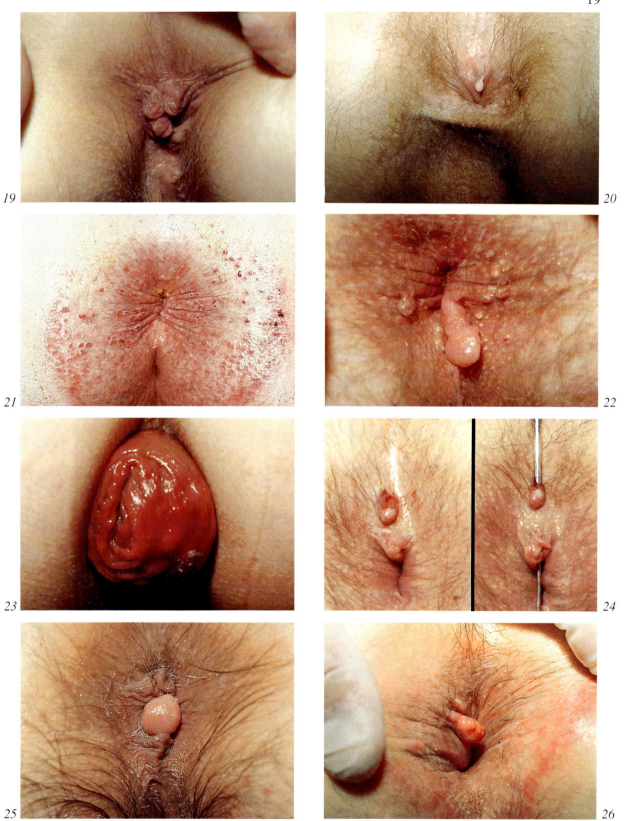

FIGURES 19–26

Left to right: skin tag (sentinel pile), lipoma, acute eczema, fibroma, complete rectal prolapse (procidentia), fistula-in-ano (right: with probe inserted into lumen), prolapsed hypertrophied anal papilla, inflamed sentinel pile.

Digital Examination

Before beginning the procedure, one should explain it to the patient. The digital examination of the rectum is best performed with the patient in the knee-elbow position. The buttocks are gently spread and the perianal region is palpated. The index finger, which is protected by a fingerstall, is then lubricated and inserted into the anus. By rotating the finger through a full circle, the anal canal and then the rectum are carefully palpated. In this way the tone of the sphincter muscles can be assessed and tumors in the anus and lower rectum can be detected. Hemorrhoids usually cannot be felt: Only fibrotic or thrombosed internal piles that are hard or painful can be detected. Hypertrophied anal papillae are sometimes mistaken for hemorrhoids, pessaries, or rings, while scybala are occasionally diagnosed as rectum tumors.

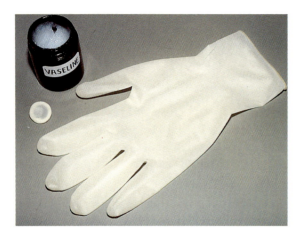

FIGURE 27
Equipment for digital examination: plastic glove, rubber fingerstall, water-soluble lubricant or vaseline.

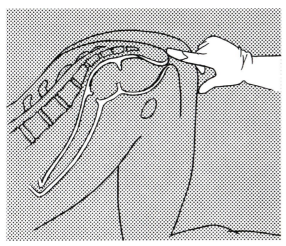

FIGURE 28
Palpation of the anal region.

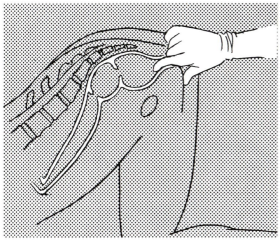

FIGURE 29
Palpating the anal canal while rotating the finger.

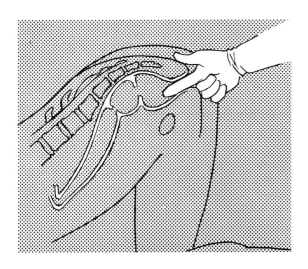

FIGURE 30
Palpation of the rectal ampulla.

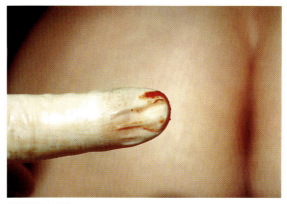

FIGURE 31
Bright red blood on the examining finger indicates a source of bleeding in the terminal colon if anal diseases are excluded.

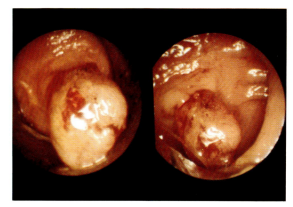

FIGURE 32
Endoscopy reveals a bleeding cherry-sized polyp at 15 cm.

Endoscopic Examination

The endoscopic examination, which consists of anoscopy and recto-sigmoidoscopy, is best performed with the patient in the knee-chest position. Following the digital examination, which slightly dilates the sphincter, the lubricated anoscope is introduced through the anal canal; with the distal end describing a downward arc, the instrument is passed under the coccyx and into the rectum. It is then slowly withdrawn while the the anal canal is viewed. The rectooscope is inserted through the anal canal in the same manner. The obturator is then removed and the instrument is inserted further into the rectum under direct vision with gentle inflation with air to aid in passing the instrument. Too much air can cause gut spasms. The rectoscope is withdrawn with a rocking motion so that every corner of the intestine can be inspected.

If a reasonable cause of the patient's complaints cannot be found by proctoscopy, then the rest of the colon must be examined by fiberoptic endoscopy and/or by radiography (barium enema, double contrast) [275].

An empty colon is a prerequisite for a meticulous endoscopic examination. Small amounts of fecal matter can be removed with long cotton swabs [9, 13, 25, 41, 63, 89, 92, 93, 100, 112, 171, 249].

Rectoscopy can be performed on more than half of all outpatients without special preparation. Laxatives may cause additional mucosal irritation, which can lead to the erroneous diagnosis of proctitis. One or two administrations of a disposable enema directly in the rectum or through the proctoscope as a high enema are usually sufficient for removing stool remaining in the rectum and the sigmoid colon [45]. Only rarely is it necessary to resort to laxatives. If fiberoptic coloscopy is planned, intensive purging with irritant laxatives and saline cathartics is recommended.

Hemorrhoids, proctitis, hypertrophied and inflamed anal papillae, anal cryptitis, polyps, and malignancies can be diagnosed by anoscopy, while rectoscopy is useful for detecting melanosis coli as well as inflammatory and infiltrative processes—two-thirds of all cancers of the large intestine are within the reach of the 30 cm long rectoscope. Rectoscopy is an examination technique that can be performed without extensive practice, whereas flexible sigmoidoscopy requires experience. In 75% of all cases, the rigid rectoscope can be used without problems, while the rest can be examined with the flexible 60–70 cm long fiberoptic endoscope.

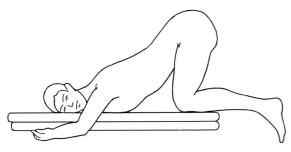

FIGURE 33
Knee-chest position.

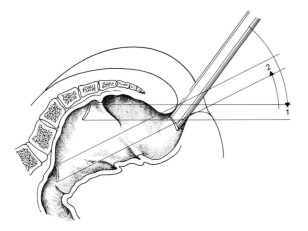

FIGURE 34
Sequence of motions for introducing the proctoscope: Blind introduction into the anal canal with simultaneous lowering of the distal end to position 1. Passage through the anal canal into the rectum while slightly elevating the distal end to position 2.

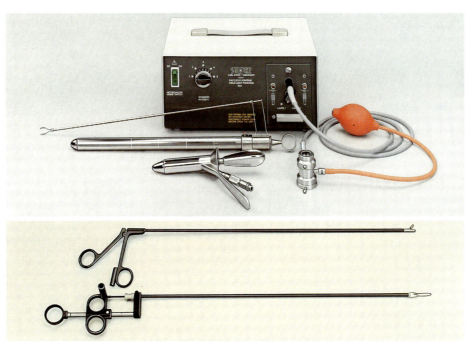

FIGURE 35
Instruments for endoscopy: Cold-light source with fiberglass light conductor to the anoscope (6–10 cm long) and the rectoscope (30 cm long, both with 20 mm diameter). Cap with viewing port, rubber bulb for inflation, and holder for cotton swabs. Lower picture: Biopsy forceps and electroresection loop.

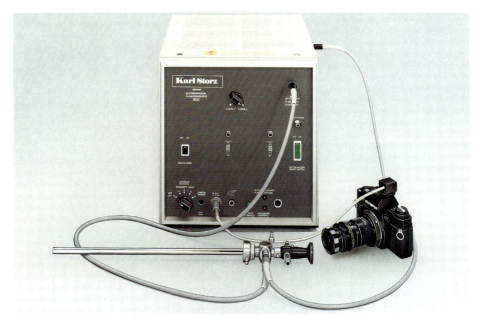

FIGURE 36
Photographic equipment for the Storz rectoscope for documentation of endoscopic findings: variable intensity electronic flash with lens system (manufactured by Karl Storz, D-7200 Tuttlingen, Germany).

Proctoscopy

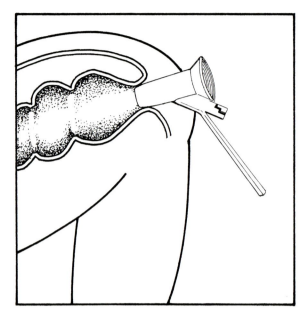

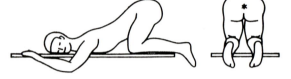

FIGURE 37
Endoscopic examination. Left: knee-chest position; right: anoscope in the anal canal.

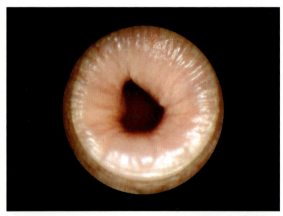

FIGURE 38
Normal pale pink anal mucosa with radial folds.

FIGURE 39
Reddish, slightly protruding, radial internal hemor-rhoids with bluish hemorrhoidal thrombosis visible through the mucosa.

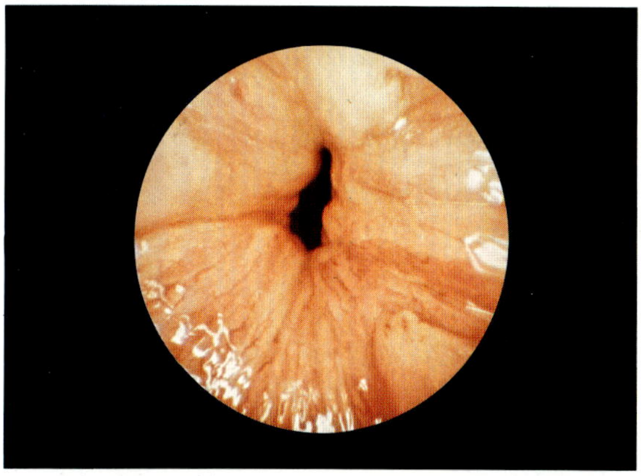

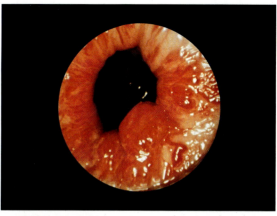

FIGURE 40
Pale pink mucosa with delicate vascularisation.

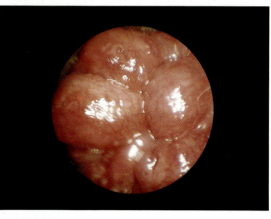

FIGURE 41
Internal hemorrhoids: tortuous vessels with nodular
protruding hemorrhoidal vessels.

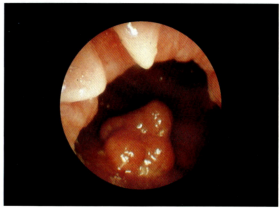

FIGURE 42
Hemorrhoidal masses protruding into the endo-
scope.

FIGURE 43
Two dorsally located, whitish, pointed hypertrophied
anal papillae. Adenoma situated ventrally in the rec-
tum which was palpated on digital examination.

Rectoscopy

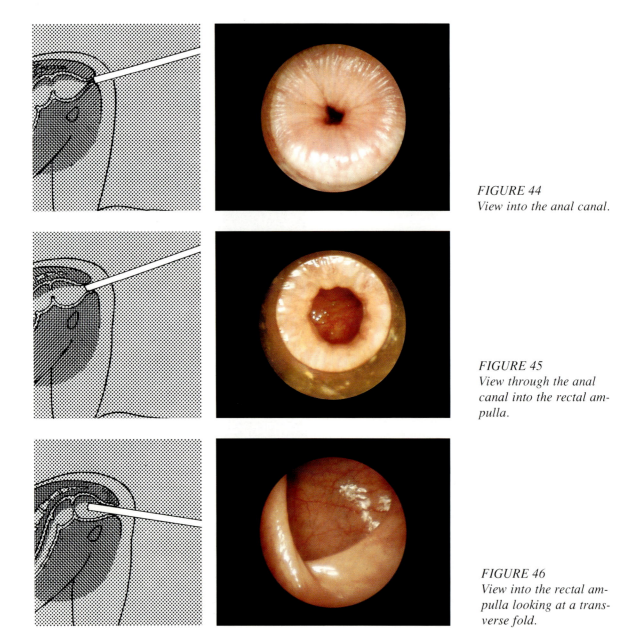

FIGURE 44
View into the anal canal.

FIGURE 45
View through the anal canal into the rectal ampulla.

FIGURE 46
View into the rectal ampulla looking at a transverse fold.

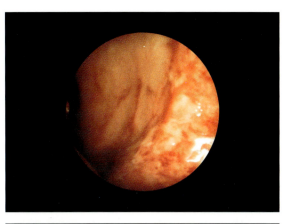

FIGURE 47
Transition from swollen, edematous, erythematous mucosa to normal mucosa with prominent vascularisation in proctitis.

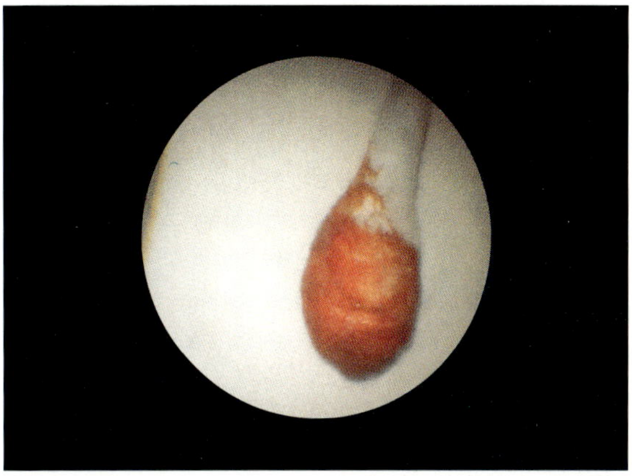

FIGURE 48
Blood on cotton swab after touching the mucosa in ulcerative colitis.

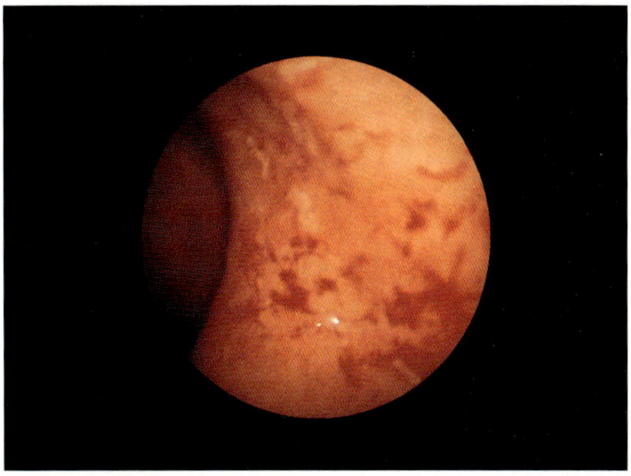

FIGURE 49
Sanguinous exudation in ulcerative colitis.

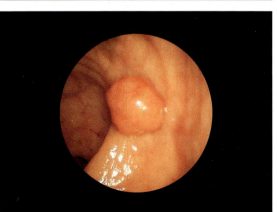

FIGURE 50
Papillomatous adenoma.

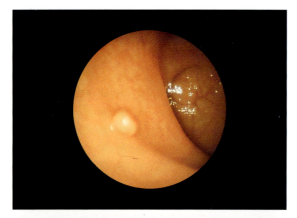

FIGURE 51
Pea-sized adenoma viewed from above.

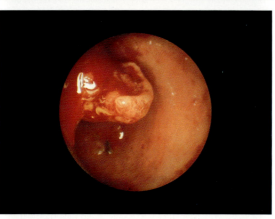

FIGURE 52
Villous adenoma.

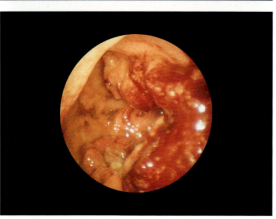

FIGURE 53
Plum-sized sesside rectal carcinoma.

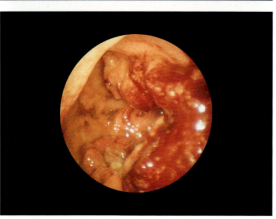

FIGURE 54
Extensive ulcerated rectal carcinoma.

Hemorrhoids

The hemorrhoidal plexus is visible directly under the external anoderm. It is congested during straining and appears as a ring of bulging livid nodules, which are soft to the touch and collapse under pressure. These are often referred to as external hemorrhoids. Thrombosis can occur in these causing painful lumps.

The internal hemorrhoidal plexus, which lies in the submucosa proximal to the pectinate line, is often referred to as internal hemorrhoids. It consists of thin-walled, mucosa-covered, large-diameter arteriovenous vascular convolutions partitioned by delicate septa; they are referred to as corpus cavernosum vecti. The plexus is fed by three branches of the superior rectal artery. Internal piles develop at the entry points of the arteries, which are situated at 3, 7 and 11 o'clock (patient in dorsal position). The venous blood drains from the plexus through the internal sphincter into the internal rectal vein. Impaired venous drainage and arterial hyperemia causes congestion of the corpus cavernosum recti. Venous drainage can be obstructed by spasms of the anal sphincter, by tumors in the true pelvis, and by habitual straining at defecation as in chronic constipation. Arterial inflow is said to be increased by increased splanchnic blood flow following copious meals, excessive alcohol consumption, rectal tumors, or by hormonal alterations during pregnancy or menstruation [94, 132, 180, 227, 228, 249].

The most common symptoms of hemorrhoids are the passage of bright red blood, burning sensations in the anus, aching or sharp perianal pain, and itching. Large hemorrhoids cause a feeling of incomplete defecation with defecation urge, sensation of foreign body in the rectum as well as incontinence. Bleeding can occur during or after defecation. It can be so slight that only traces are seen on the toilet paper, or it can be so massive that it spatters the entire toilet bowl. The vascular lesions usually close immediately and can only rarely be found on subsequent anoscopy.

Large internal hemorrhoids may be palpated as soft cushions, having a somewhat firmer consistency when fibrotic or thrombosed. The diagnosis is confirmed by anoscopy. Tortuous reddish vessels are visible through the anoscope; these become more prominent when venous efflux is prevented by compression with the tip of the instrument. In hyperplasia of the corpus cavernosum recti, they protrude into the endoscope. Straining can cause them to prolapse into the anoscope, especially at the entry points of the branches of the superior rectal artery; that is, at 3, 7 and 11 o'clock.

Hemorrhoids are classified in four degrees:

- First-degree hemorrhoids are visible on anoscopy as reddish lumps protruding into the anoscope on straining.

- Second-degree hemorrhoids prolapse through the anal canal but return spontaneously.

- Third-degree hemorrhoids require manual replacement.

- If replacement is no longer possible, one refers to them as fourth-degree hemorrhoids [11, 25, 34, 77, 182, 194, 195, 221, 222, 249, 262, 263, 264] (cf. Figure 100).

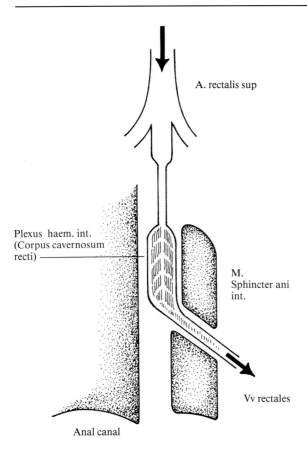

A. rectalis sup

Plexus haem. int.
(Corpus cavernosum
recti)

M.
Sphincter ani
int.

Vv rectales

Anal canal

FIGURE 55
Diagram of the internal rectal plexus (corpus caver-
nosum recti).

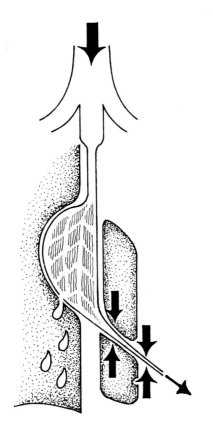

Increased arterial supply and/or impaired venous
drainage (anal spasm, increased intraabdominal
pressure) cause hyperplasia of the corpus caverno-
sum. Bright red blood comes from mucosal tears
during defecation.

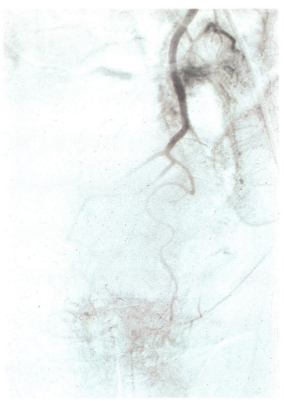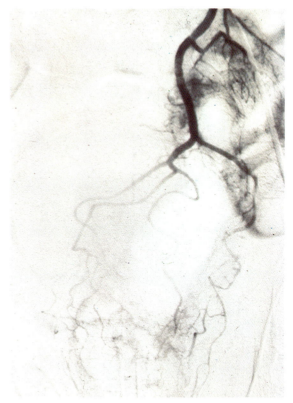

FIGURE 56
Left: Selective arteriography of the superior rectal artery.
Right: Contrast medium in pools of the internal hemorrhoidal plexus (Corpus cavernosum recti).

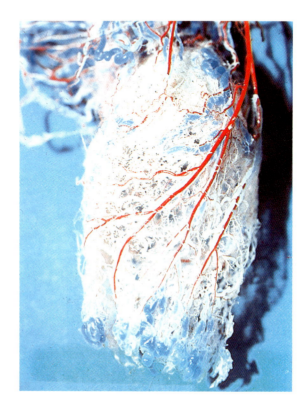

FIGURE 57
Resin corrosion cast of rectal vessels: Intraarterial and intravenous of resin after fixation with chromic acid. The delicate radicles of the red superior rectal artery connect with the dilated blue vessels of the internal venous plexus (corpus cavernosum recti).
Figures 56 and 57 were provided by Dr. E. Parnaud of the Département de Proctologie, Hôpital des Diaconesses in Paris.

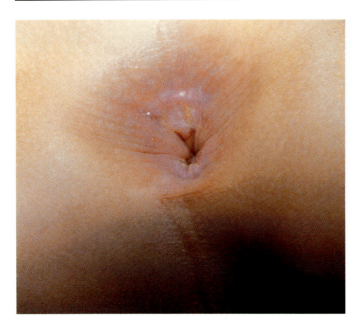

FIGURE 58
Bluish ring of the inferior venous plexus
(external hemorrhoidal plexus).

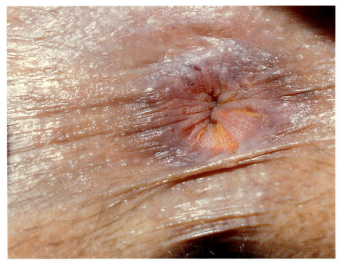

FIGURE 59
The inferior venous plexus is visible as a
bluish ring after spreading the folds of the
perianal skin.

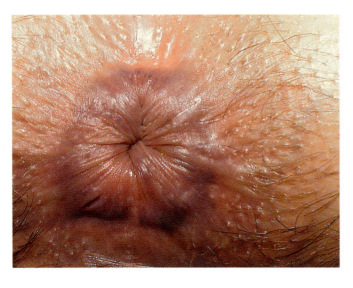

FIGURE 60
The inferior venous plexus bulges during
straining.

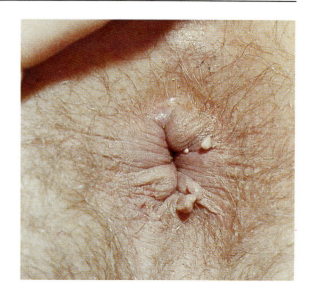

FIGURE 61
Three fibromas seen after spreading the perianal skin.

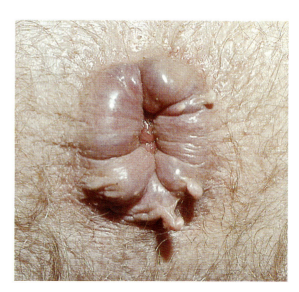

FIGURE 62
During straining, the inferior venous plexus protrudes as a bluish circular mass. The boundry between perianal skin and anoderm is seen as a corona at the level of the three fibromas.

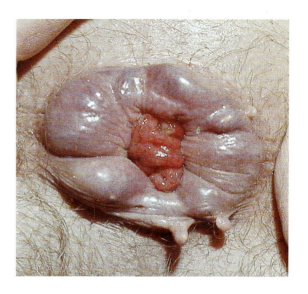

FIGURE 63
At maximal straining, a partial mucosal prolapse appears, which can be recognized by the bright red mucous membrane.

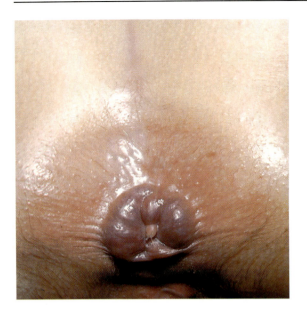

FIGURE 64
Circular, massively engorged inferior venous plexus with a paler hypertrophied anal papilla protruding at the center.

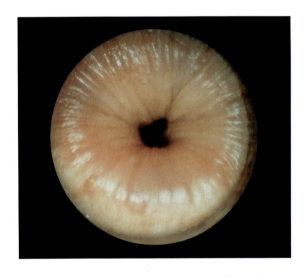

FIGURE 65
Normal pale-pink, smooth, shiny, radially folded mucosa of the anal canal.

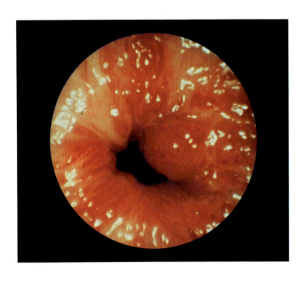

FIGURE 66
Radiating, red, slightly prominent and tortuous internal hemorrhoids.

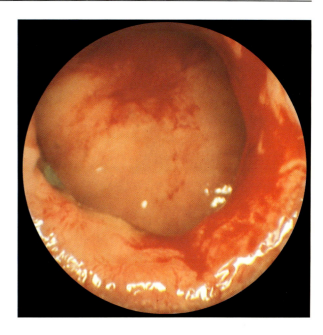

FIGURE 67
Bleeding hemorrhoids.

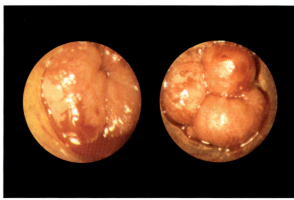

FIGURE 68
During anoscopy, there are bleeding internal hemorrhoids which protrude into the anoscope at right posterior, right anterior and left lateral on straining. These are designated as first-degree hemorrhoids.

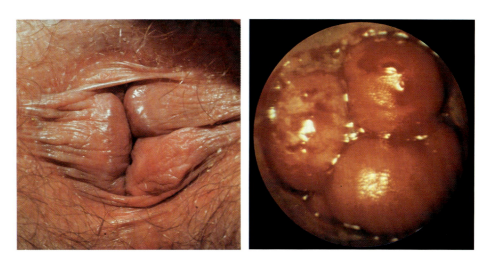

FIGURES 69 & 70
Second-degree hemorrhoids: Straining causes the anoderm to bulge at 2, 5, and 9 o'clock. At endoscopy, one finds prolapsing hemorrhoidal masses in the corresponding positions.

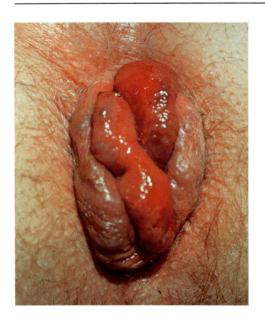

FIGURE 71
Prolapsed, reducible hemorrhoids at 2, 5, and 9 o'clock in knee-chest position (third-degree hemorrhoids).

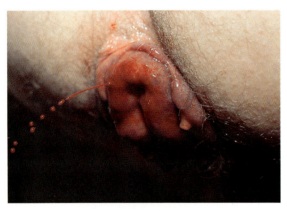

FIGURE 72
Prolapsed, actively bleeding, reducible hemorrhoidal masses (third-degree hemorrhoids).

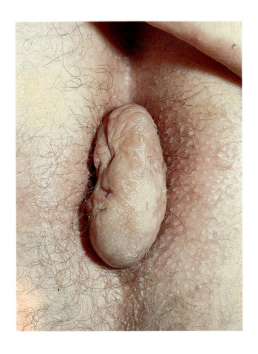

FIGURE 73
Prolapsed hemorrhoids that cannot be replaced in the anal canal (fourth-degree hemorrhoids).

Treatment of Hemorrhoids

Treatment of the symptoms of hemorrhoids, such as itching, burning, pain, and bloody or mucous discharge begins with good anal hygiene and regulation of bowel habits. The anal region is cleansed with water to which chamomile can be added as desired. Soap is not used. The stool should be kept soft. Constipation can be treated with a high-residue diet, ample fluid intake, and bulk laxatives. With diarrhea, laxative foods and beverages such as cabbage, sauerkraut, apple or orange juice should be avoided. Suppositories can bring rapid relief. To achieve maximal effect on the anal mucosa, the patient should be instructed to keep the suppository in the anal canal for at least 1 or 2 minutes before it is passed completely into the rectal ampulla. The dilators included with many brands of hemorrhoid salves are also very useful. With them it is possible to relieve a sphincter spasm, thus improving venous drainage. In cases of highly inflamed hemorrhoids or fissures, however, the use of a dilator may be painful. Applying the ointment with the finger is usually better tolerated.

Local application of warmth with a heated tube is usually perceived as agreeable: The sphincter is relaxed and venous drainage is facilitated.

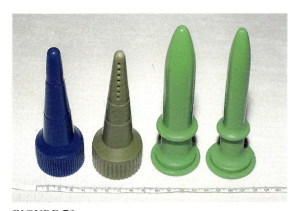

FIGURE 73a
Dilators.

If these measures are not successful within 2 weeks, sclero-therapy is recommended [5, 10, 11, 19, 23, 25, 28, 47, 50, 94, 113, 134, 139, 150, 153, 158, 161, 165, 166, 247, 249, 257].

Sclero-Therapy

Injection Therapy

The aim of sclero-therapy is to achieve hemostasis by cicatricial fixation of the hemorrhoidal vessels and by reduction of their blood supply. This is done by applying an irritant stimulus to the mucosa above the hemorrhoid, which induces a local inflammatory tissue reaction leading to cicatricial contraction with constriction of the afferent vessels. This stimulus can be thermal, as in electrocoagulation [72], cryosurgery, or infrared coagulation, or chemical following injection of irritant preparations. The most common methods of chemical sclero-therapy are those described by Blond [18] and Bensaude [10]. In Blond's method, an angled needle and an anoscope with side opening are used to inject single drops of the sclerosant under the mucosa around the entire circumference. Six to eight sessions are usually necessary to stop bleeding from the hemorrhoids.

In the method described by Bensaude, the sclerosant is injected at an acute angle into the submucosa above the hemorrhoids. The deposit causes a small bulge, which is paler than the neighboring mucosa (Figure 85). Injections that are too superficial often cause bleeding from mucosal necrosis, while those that are placed too deep in the muscular layers can cause severe pain. Two injections on opposite sides of the rectum are given at weekly intervals in the sequence shown in Figure 86. The entire treatment takes three to four sessions, which may be repeated if necessary after 4 to 6 weeks.

Commonly used sclerosants are sodium iodide, iodine, and benzyl alcohol, quinine-urethan, phenol in almond oil and a 1% solution of polidocanol.

Acute inflammatory or thrombotic disorders, pregnancy, severe hypertension, or coagulation disorders are contraindications for sclero-therapy.

The most common complication is mucosal necrosis with bleeding. Secondary hemorrhage after sclero-therapy can take on life-threatening dimensions and therefore always warrants a careful endoscopic examination. Necrosis is normally limited (Figures 87 and 88), although in rare cases there is extensive tissue destruction. This is probably because of an allergic reaction to the sclerosant. This complication is avoided by methods of sclero-therapy, such as electrocoagulation, cryotherapy, or infrared coagulation, which do not rely on the injection of foreign material [33, 86, 93, 170, 239, 249, 255].

Infrared Coagulation (Photocoagulation)

The beam of infrared light induces an inflammatory reaction in the mucosa with cicatricial contraction and vascular narrowing.

Method: The hemorrhoids are visualized by anoscopy, and the stimulus is applied to the mucosa directly above the hemorrhoid (Figure 93). The tip of the light conductor in placed in direct contact with the mucosa. The built-in timer is set to limit each exposure to one second. The beam is triggered by a switch in the handgrip. The probe is covered with a sapphire tip that allows infrared light to pass without attenuation. Because of its hydrophobic properties, the tip does not adhere to tissue after coagulation; this distinguishes it from electrocoagulation and prevents the mucosa from tearing when the tip is withdrawn. The treated site is visible as a circumscribed grayish area. After one week a slight retraction can still be discerned which has a reddish hue because of the newly sprouting capillaries. Two weeks later, only a discrete cicatricial retraction remains which is covered by normal mucosa and disappears after a further one to two weeks. Two sessions with four coagulation sites each usually stop hemorrhoidal bleeding. In the first session the tip is applied at 3, 6, 9, and 12 o'clock, and in the following at 2, 4, 8, and 10 o'clock. Six to eight sessions are necessary to eradicate prolapsed hemorrhoids.

The heat is unpleasant for some patients. Slight bleeding may occur from the edges of the heat-induced ulcerations. Significant blood loss occurs only if the tip is applied directly to the hemorrhoid and not above it [4, 33, 101, 103, 110, 111, 126, 147, 157, 164, 170, 181, 213, 241, 260].

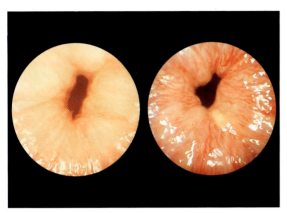

FIGURE 74
Left: normal mucosa with pale-pink color and radial folds; right: tortuous, red hemorrhoidal vessels.

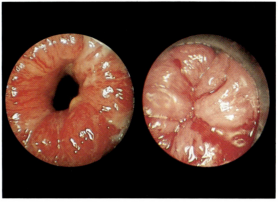

FIGURE 75
Endoscopic view of bleeding internal hemorrhoids.

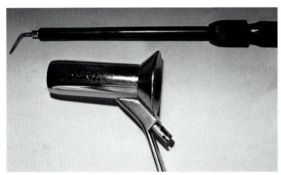

FIGURE 76
Instruments used for electrocoagulation: Bent needle attached to extension piece with handgrip and anoscope.

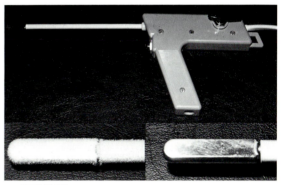

FIGURE 78
Cryotherapy pistol. Below right: metal tip; left: covered with ice after cooling to –90 °C.

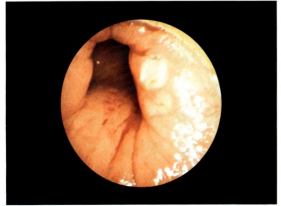

FIGURE 77
Grayish mucosa after electrocoagulation.

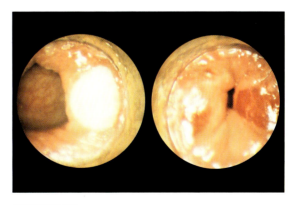

FIGURE 79
Left: the frozen area immediately after treatment; right: five minutes later this appears as a red spot.

Sclerosing injection by the method of Blond

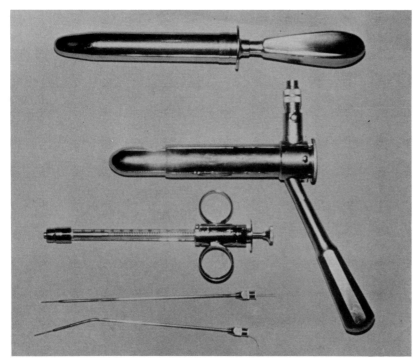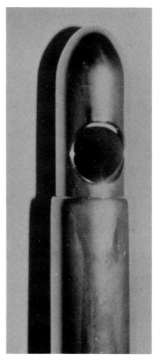

FIGURES 80 & 81
Instruments for sclerosing hemorrhoids by the method of Blond. Anoscope tube with a side-opening; disassembled in mandrin and tube, needles with straight and angled tips.

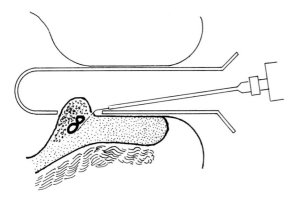

FIGURE 82
Submucosal injection of hemorrhoids.

Sclerosing injection by the method of Bensaude

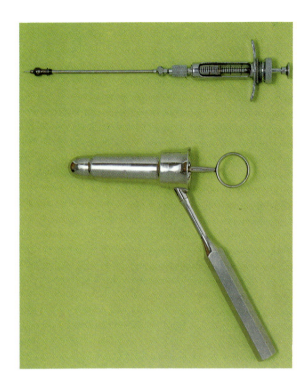

FIGURE 83
Instruments for sclerosing hemorrhoids by the method of Bensaude: Rotatable anoscope with beveled end, syringe with connecting piece and 5–6 mm long needle.

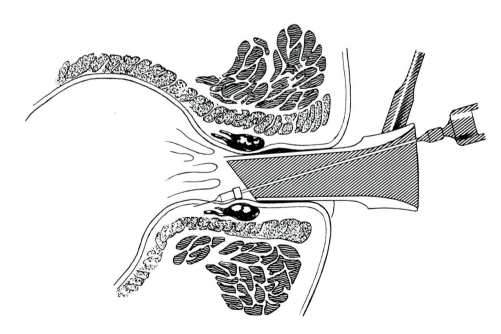

FIGURE 84
The needle is inserted at an acute angle into the submucosa above the hemorrhoid, and 0.5–1 ml of the sclerosant is injected.

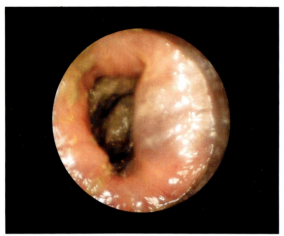

FIGURE 85
Pale bulging mucosa after injecting the sclerosant at 3 o'clock.

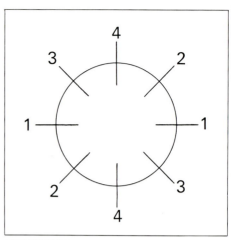

FIGURE 86
Sequence of sclerosant injections (two injections at each session).

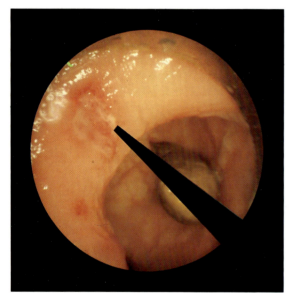

FIGURE 87
Limited necrosis after injection of sclerosant.

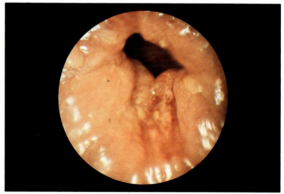

FIGURE 88
Limited necrosis in the anterior midline after injecting sclerosant.

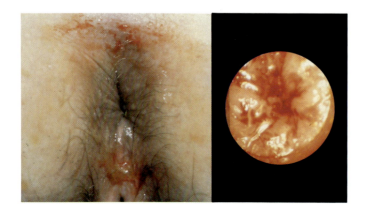

FIGURE 89
Bleeding hemorrhoids are an indication for photocoagulation. Traces of blood are seen around the anus, and endoscopy reveals bleeding internal hemorrhoids.

Infrared coagulation

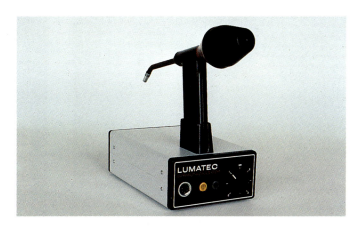

FIGURE 90
Infrared coagulator with power supply and time switch. Manufactured by Lumatec GmbH, Steinerstr. 15, D-8000 München 70, Germany.

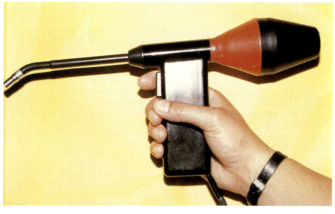

FIGURE 91
Pistol-shaped infrared coagulator held with the index finger on the trigger.

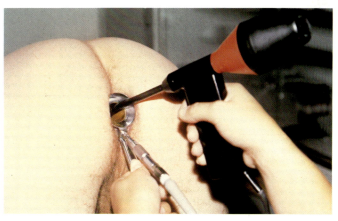

FIGURE 92
The hemorrhoids are visualized with the anoscope and the light conductor is inserted through the lumen.

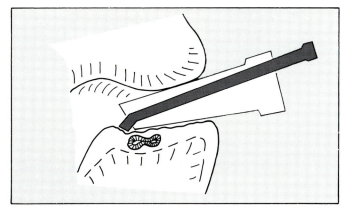

FIGURE 93
The infrared light is applied above the piles.

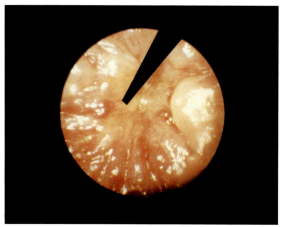

FIGURE 94
The site for coagulation is chosen under direct vision directly above the hemorrhoid mass.

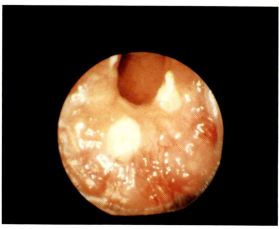

FIGURE 95
The action of the infrared beam leaves a circumscribed, grayish spot on the mucosa.

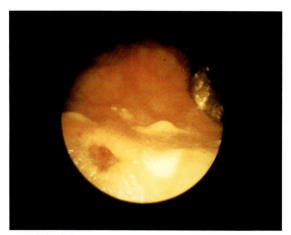

FIGURE 96
After one week a slightly retracted area is found whose reddish color comes from newly sprouting capillaries.

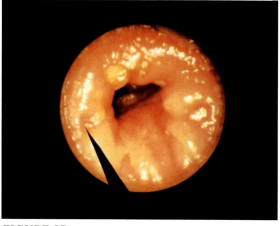

FIGURE 97
Two weeks later only an inconspicuous scarred dimple can be seen.

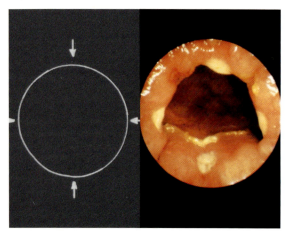

FIGURE 98
The four sites that have been coagulated.

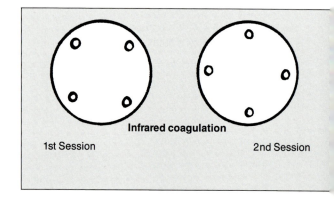

FIGURE 99
Schematic representation of the sites to which infrared coagulation is applied.

Rubber-Band Ligation for Treatment of Prolapsing Hemorrhoids

Prolapsing second- or third-degree hemorrhoids are effectively treated by rubber-band ligation. The prolapsed piles are ligated at their pedicle with a rubber band. The ligature is applied above the pectinate line in the insensitive region of the anal canal and is therefore usually painless. The hemorrhoids are visualized through the anoscope, grasped with forceps or by suction, and pulled into a tube around which the rubber band has been stretched. This is then slipped over the pile, ligating it at its pedicle. After 5 to 7 days the pile mass undergoes necrosis and sloughs off leaving a small ulcer. Only rarely does secondary arterial bleeding occur before the ulcer is completely healed. The patients should be informed about this possibility and instructed to return for examination if the bleeding is profuse. Pain is a further complication occurring either immediately after ligation, if the band is applied too low, or delayed as a result of sphincter muscle spasm. Immediate pain is treated by cutting the rubber band with scissors and removing it. Pain from a spasm of the anal canal usually responds to analgesics, although local anesthesia is occasionally necessary to stop the painful contractions. Prolapsed hemorrhoids can be ligated directly without the anoscope [7, 8, 25, 33, 122, 143, 144, 155, 249].

FIGURE 100

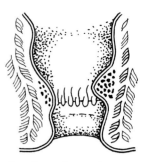

Hemorrhoid mass prolapsing into the endoscope (first-degree hemorrhoids).

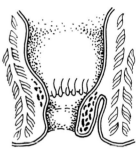

Hemorrhoid prolapsing through the anus, which slides back spontaneously (second-degree hemorrhoids).

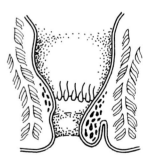

Hemorrhoid that must be replaced manually (third-degree hemorrhoids).

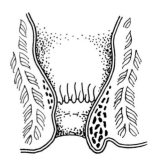

Permanently prolapsed hemorrhoid (fourth-degree hemorrhoids).

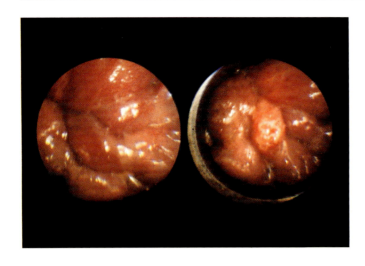

FIGURE 101
Hemorrhoids bulging into the anoscope (first degree hemorrhoids).

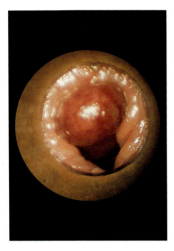
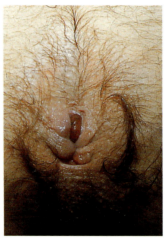

FIGURE 102a
Small prolapsed hemorrhoids. They appear during straining and slide back spontaneously (second-degree hemorrhoids).

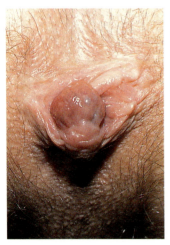
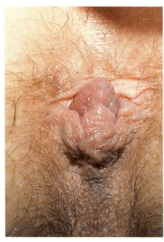

FIGURE 102b
Prolapsed hemorrhoids. They appear after defection and do not slide back spontaneously (third-degree hemorrhoids).

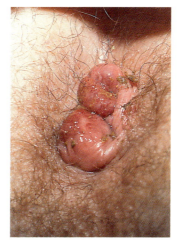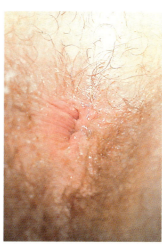

FIGURE 103
*Prolapsed hemorrhoids that must be re-
duced manually (third-degree hemorrhoid).*

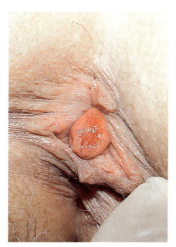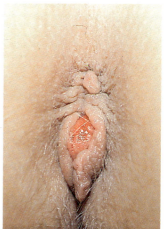

FIGURE 104
*Prolapsed hemorrhoids that must be re-
duced manually (third-degree hemorrhoid).*

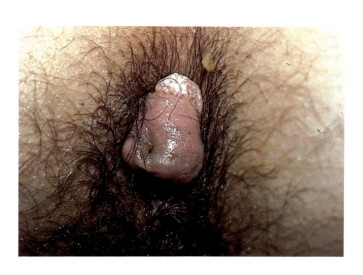

FIGURE 105
*Prolapsed hemorrhoids with external at-
tachment that can no longer be replaced
(fourth-degree hemorrhoid).*

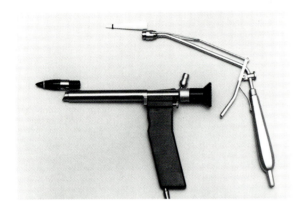

FIGURE 106
Apparatus for rubber-band ligation of prolapsing hemorrhoids. Cone for fitting rubber bands. Suction ligation instrument and vacuum ligation anoscope (Treier Endoskopie AG, CH-6215 Beromünster, Switzerland).

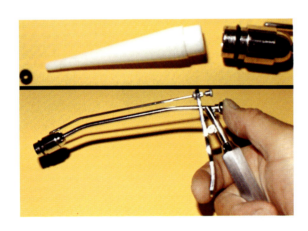

FIGURE 107
Using the teflon cone, the rubber band is stretched over the metal cylinder. The suction valve is closed with the thumb. The band is slipped off by a mechanism operated by the index finger.

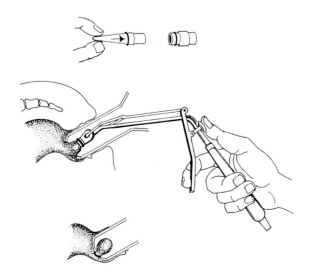

FIGURE 108
The prolapsed hemorrhoid is suctioned into the metal tube and the rubber band is slipped over it. Below: Ligated pile

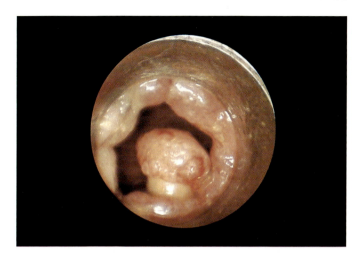

FIGURE 109
Ligated pile: a white rubber band is visible at the pedicle.

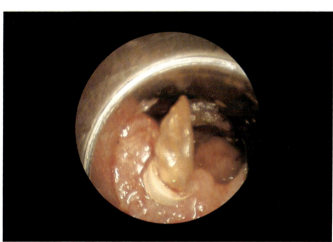

FIGURE 110
Necrotic pile 7 days after ligation.

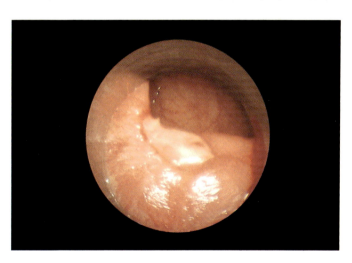

FIGURE 111
A whitish area remains in the mucosa after the necrotic hemorrhoid has sloughed off.

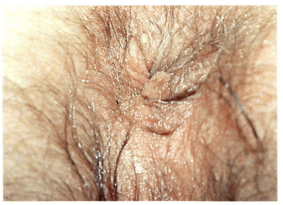
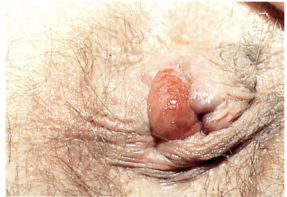

112

113

FIGURES 112 & 113
Large reddish mass protruding through the anus during straining (second-degree hemorrhoid) which can be ligated externally.

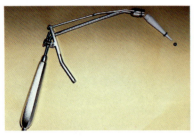
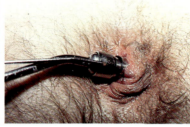
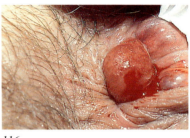

114

115

116

FIGURES 114–116
Suction ligation instrument with a metal cylinder at the distal end. The rubber band is stretched onto the cylinder using the teflon cone. The prolapsed hemorrhoid is drawn by suction into the metal cylinder. A sliding cylinder then pushes the stretched rubber band off the tube over the mass, ligating it at its pedicle.

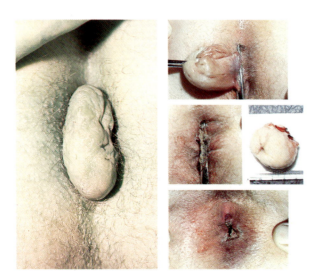

FIGURE 117
Prolapsed fourth-degree hemorrhoid. A large smooth mass covered with skin is situated directly outside the anus. Under anesthesia, the base of the mass is clamped with a Kocher's forceps, and the mass is then resected along the clamp with scissors. The resection site is cauterized with the infrared coagulator before the clamp is removed. The wound is treated with panthenol creams.

Surgical Treatment

Extensive prolapsing or externally fixed hemorrhoids are treated surgically either by the method of Milligan and Morgan, or by that introduced by Parks [33, 79, 83, 137, 172, 189, 276]. The method of circular hemorrhoidectomy described by Whitehouse should no longer be used since it can cause anal narrowing or incontinence with mucosal prolapse (Figures 123–126). Healing is reported to be more rapid when a laser is used for excision instead of a scalpel [42, 50, 215, 249, 265]. Cryosurgery, on the other hand, is associated with more extensive edema formation and extremely annoying secretions [43, 119, 214, 278].

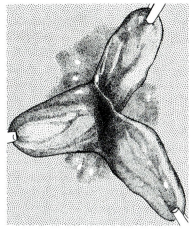

FIGURE 119
Hemorrhoidectomy described by Milligan and Morgan (patient in knee-chest position). The three main masses at 2, 5, and 9 o'clock are grasped with forceps and drawn outwards.

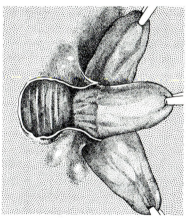

FIGURE 120
Each mass is pulled medially, mobilised with a semicircular perianal incision and dissected free down to its vascular pedicle in the anal canal. The pedicle is transfixed and ligated and the piles are excised.

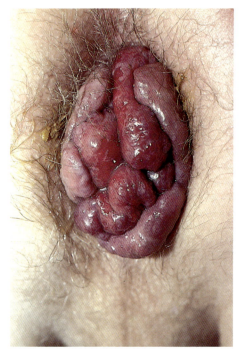

FIGURE 118
Extensive prolapsed hemorrhoids for which surgical therapy is indicated.

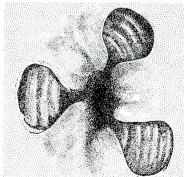

FIGURE 121
After excision of the three main masses with three skin bridges and the internal sphincter visible at the floor of the wound.

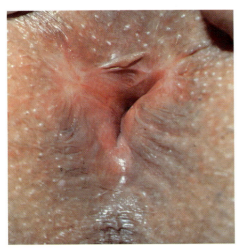

FIGURE 122
After the Milligan-Morgan operation: normal scar tissue can be seen separted by bridges of anoderm.

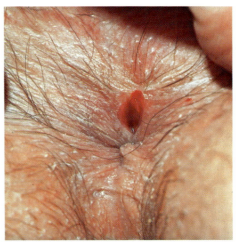

FIGURE 123
Cicatrical narrowing following a Whitehead operation.

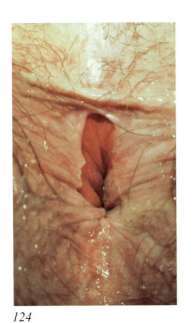

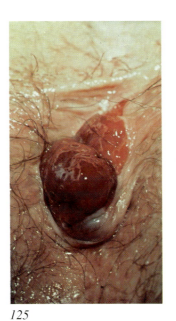

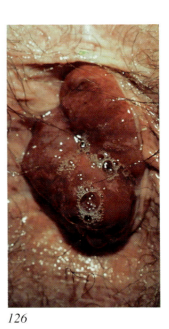

124 *125* *126*

FIGURES 124–126
Mucosal prolapse following Whitehead operation: The hemorrhoids are removed by circumferential excision and the mucosa is sutured to the perianal skin. During straining, the mucosa of the rectum protrudes first left posteriorly and then anteriorly on the right.

Diseases Associated with Hemorrhoids

Inflammation of internal hemorrhoids can spread to adjacent tissue leading to proctitis with hyperemic rectal mucosa, irritation of the anal glands with hypersecretion and anal mucous discharge, which, in turn, can cause periproctitis and anal eczema.

Spread of the inflammation from the internal hemorrhoids via marginal vessels can cause thrombophlebitis of the external subcutaneous venous plexus; a painful condition known as acute thrombotic external piles. A skin tag often remains after healing under which stool can be retained and cause inflammation of the anal mucosa. This can tear during defecation leading to an anal fissure.

Inflammatory processes in the anal canal can spread to the papillae and crypts, causing papillitis and anal cryptitis. These can persist and lead to abscesses or a fistula-in-ano.

The next pages discuss the following:

– Proctitis

– Periproctitis

– Anal cryptitis

– Anal papillitis

– Thrombosed external hemorrhoids (external anal thrombosis)

– Fissure-in-ano

– Fistula-in-ano

– Anal abscess

Proctitis

Proctitis may be caused by the spread of inflammation from hemorrhoids to the anal mucosa. Symptoms include pruritus, especially after defecation, and serous secretions from the hyperemic mucosa which soil the underwear. Endoscopy reveals a erythematous or purplish mucosa, engorged vessels, transient mucosal abrasions, or even ulceration. Predisposing factors are taking hot spices, coffee and chocolate as well as alcohol abuse, laxatives and constipation or diarrhea. Mucoid or purulent discharge suggests gonococcal or chlamydial infection. This is confirmed by a microscopical examination of a stained smear or by culture [41, 134].

Therapy of unspecific proctitis consists of eliminating noxious exogenous agents and applying hemorrhoidal salves and suppositories. These usually bring rapid relief. Local cooling with a glycocol-filled bag that is cooled in the freezing compartment of the refrigerator also has an antiphlogistic effect [248]. The bag is lubricated with hemorrhoid jelly and inserted into the anal canal for about 5 minutes several times a day. The cold bag can sometimes cause

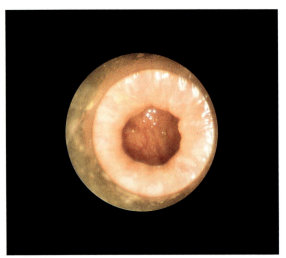

FIGURE 127
Normal anal mucosa with its pale pink color.

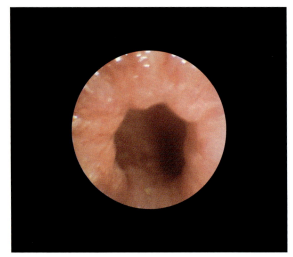

FIGURE 128
Proctitis: The mucosa is edematous and red.

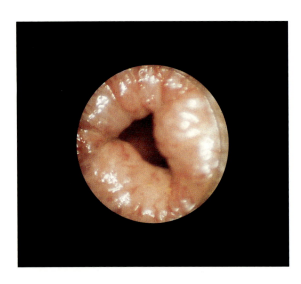

FIGURE 129
Proctitis: Purplish mucosa with a superficial abrasion.

a painful sphincter spasm. A recently developed local antiphlogistic treatment of unspecific anal and rectal inflammation is with 5-amino-salicylic acid suppositories.

Gonorrheal proctitis must be treated with penicillin. Tetracycline or oxytetracycline should be given if chlamydiae are the causative organisms (see also the chapter on sexually transmitted diseases).

Periproctitis (Perianal Dermatitis)

The secretions in proctitis may cause inflammatory changes of the perianal skin. Other causative factors are the use of newspaper for cleaning the anus, food allergies, oxyuriasis, diabetes mellitus, antibiotics, and soaps or detergents. Mycosis is fairly common. Symptoms include itching, weeping, and occasional traces of blood on the toilet paper. On inspection one finds erythematous, oozing, indurated perianal skin, often with superficial ulcerations.

Treatment aims at alleviating proctitis with hemorrhoid jelly and suppositories, or sclerotherapy, eliminating noxious exogenous agents, and treating fungal infection with antimycotics [41, 106, 160, 256, 257] (see also the chapter on eczema).

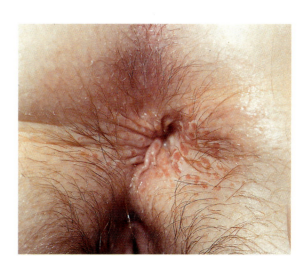

FIGURE 130
Excoriated erythematous perianal skin.

Cryptitis and Papillitis

The anal papillae are formed by proximal protuberances of the anal epithelium, which extend to and are contiguous with the mucous ridges of the anal columns. The furrowed anal epithelium between the papillae forms pockets known as crypts of Morgagni or anal sinus. These crypts terminate in the perianal glands. Both papillae and crypts are susceptible to injury and infection. The caustic liquid stools associated with diarrhea or laxatives, and the consumption of hot spices, chocolate, white wine, or coffee can lead to inflammation. Normal anal papillae are only barely visible, but when inflamed they hypertrophy and can prolapse.

Symptoms: aching pain in the anus, exacerbated by defecation. At endoscopy one finds edema, erythema, a tendency toward bleeding, and pain on palpation with a probe. Purulent matter found in the crypts should be cultured.

Therapy: If gonococcae are found, the infection must be treated with penicillin. In other cases the crypt is cut with a hooked knife (Figure 137), and the tips of the hypertrophied papillae are swabbed with silver nitrate. Hemorrhoid suppositories are used for follow-up treatment. Large, prolapsing hypertrophied papillae are removed under local anesthesia [41, 47, 50, 68, 166, 249].

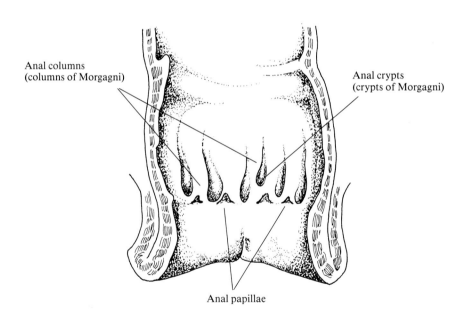

Anal columns (columns of Morgagni)

Anal crypts (crypts of Morgagni)

Anal papillae

FIGURE 131
Anatomy of the lining of the anal canal.

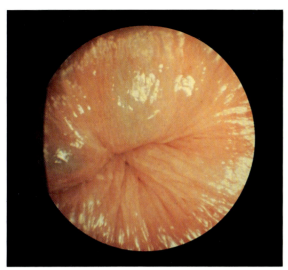

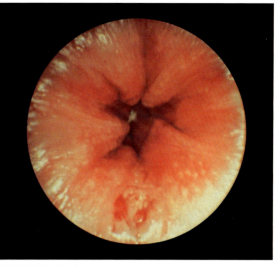

FIGURE 132

Cryptitis: Normal pale pink mucosa with a thrombosed hemorrhoid the size of a grain of rice at 9 o'clock.

FIGURE 133

The same patient as in Figure 132. When the anoscope is advanced, a red, tender crypt comes into view at 6 o'clock.

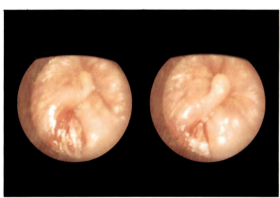

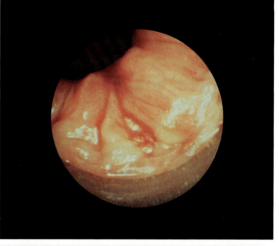

FIGURE 134

Reddened, painful crypt adjacent to a hypertrophic anal papilla in the anterior midline.

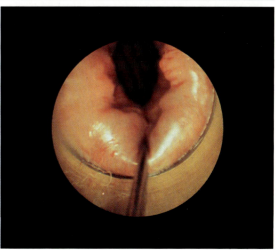

FIGURES 135 & 136

Reddened crypt in the anal canal which is tender to touch. A bent blunt probe is inserted into an internal fistula opening.

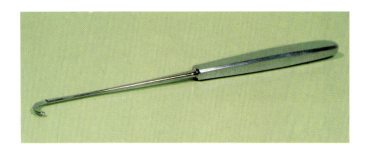

FIGURE 137
Hooked knife for opening inflamed crypts.

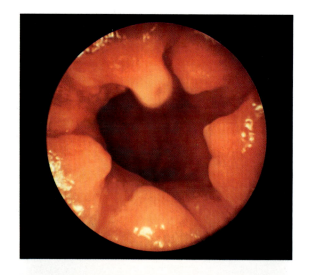

FIGURE 138
Inflamed, edematous, hypertrophic anal papilla.

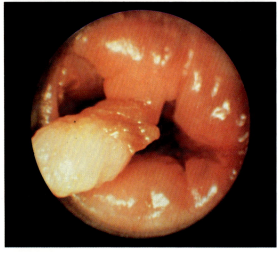

FIGURE 139
Hyperkeratotic prolapsed papilla.

FIGURE 140
Edematous, hypertrophic papillae in proctitis.

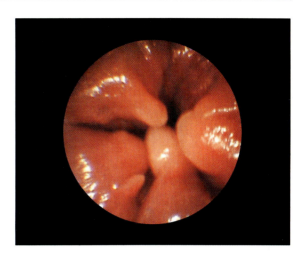

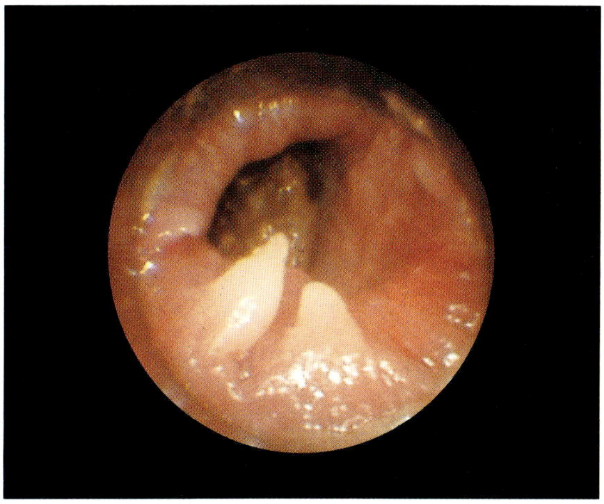

FIGURE 141
Chronic papillitis with whitish, hyperkeratotic tips on the papillae ("cat's teeth").

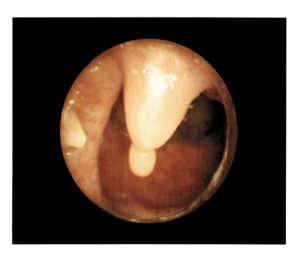

FIGURE 142
Hypertrophic papilla which can be mistaken for a hemorrhoid on digital examination.

Perianal Hematoma (acute thrombotic external piles, thrombosed external hemorrhoids, external anal thrombosis)

Inflammatory processes in the anal canal can spread to subcutaneous external venous plexus via marginal vessels causing intravascular thrombosis. Increases in intraabdominal pressure, occurring with excessive straining with constipation, heavy lifting, coughing and sneezing, and diarrhea, can cause the venous wall to rupture. Part of the blood coagulates extravascularly and forms a perianal hematoma [34, 41].

Symptoms: Lumps with a sensation of pressure and tightness. Inspection and palpation reveal a bluish mass, which is firm to the touch and painful.

Therapy: A salve containing heparin is applied in cases in which the the pain is not severe [250]. If the pain is severe, the lump can be incised with or without local anesthesia and the clot removed. Follow-up treatment is with a heparin salve. The incision should be done within the first 72 hours; thereafter, the thrombus has started to organize and is best treated conservatively. Extensive thromboses can be treated by excision of a skin flap.

In rare cases the clot is extruded spontaneously. Thrombosed hemorrhoids that are left untreated or are treated conservatively can leave skin tags. Chafing on the underwear or passage of liquid stool can cause inflammation of these tags with edematous swelling and pain. The application of chamomile compresses or ointment bring rapid relief. They can be removed under local anesthesia. The skin tags often impair anal hygiene: Stool can be retained in the folds causing maceration of the skin with eczema and fissures.

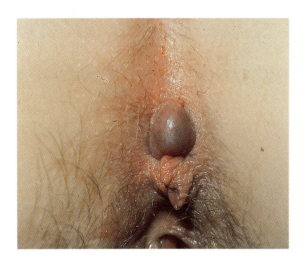

FIGURE 143
External anal thromboses on the right.

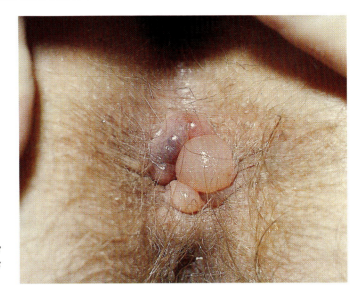

FIGURE 144
External anal thrombosis with edema of the anoderm. On the left are two bluish masses and on the right the anoderm is swollen.

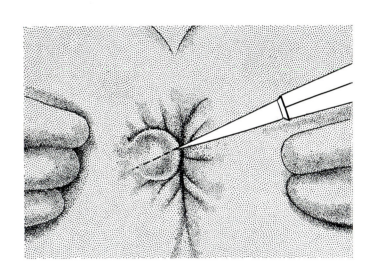

FIGURE 145
Radial incision of the hematoma.

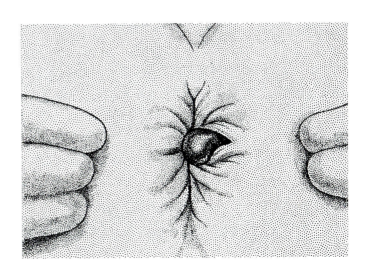

FIGURE 146
Spontaneous expulsion of the clot.

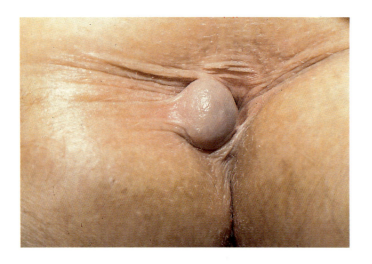

FIGURE 147
Perianal hematoma on the left.

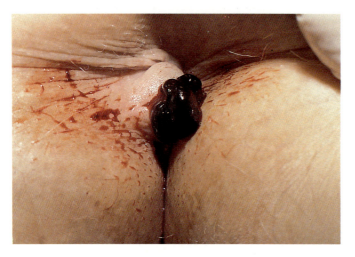

FIGURE 148
The same patient as in Figure 147 after evacuation of the clot through a radial incision.

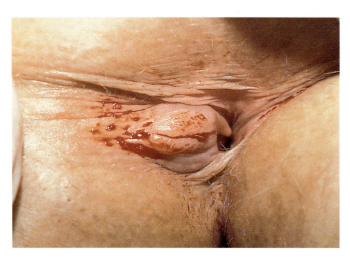

FIGURE 149
The same patient after evacuation of the clot.

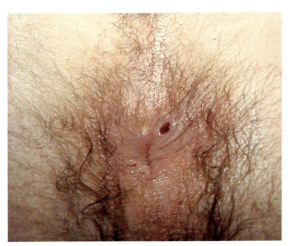

FIGURE 150
Spontaneously ruptured hematoma near the posterior midline.

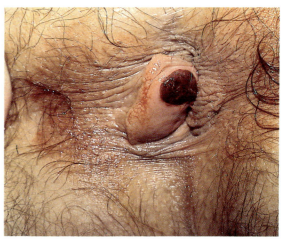

FIGURE 151
Spontaneously ruptured hematoma with skin tag.

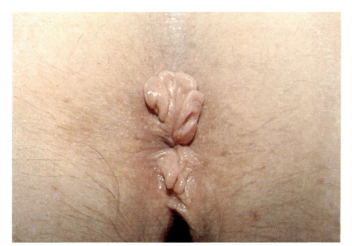

FIGURE 152
Skin tag after spontaneously healed external anal thrombosis (sentinel pile).

FIGURE 153 ➤
Red, inflamed, painful skin tag caused by mechanical irritation.

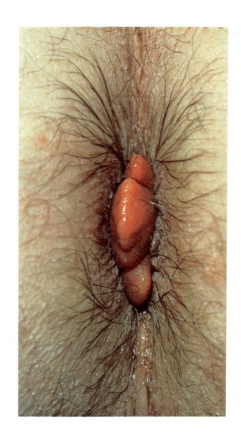

Anal Fissure
(fissura-in-ano)

An anal fissure is a tear in the anoderm which can penetrate down to the internal sphincter muscle. The tears occur at the commissures, which are the weakest points, for example, during passage of hard constipated stool [249]. A vascular cause of anal fissures is the ulceration of perianal thromboses [9, 220].

The triad of pain, bleeding, and sphincter spasm are characteristic symptoms. Pain begins during defecation or a few minutes thereafter and can persist for hours. Secondary constipation is a common consequence of the fear of defecating; this disappears rapidly, however, once the fissure has healed. The pain can become unbearable, radiating into the bladder, uterus, prostate, and thighs. The pain can be caused by walking, exertion, or coughing, and can lead to difficulties with micturition. Bleeding, dripping or freely flowing, occurs mainly during the passage of stool. The sphincter spasm is frequently so intense that digital examination is only possible after the fissure has been infiltrated with a local anesthetic (1% lignocaine).

Seventy-five percent of all anal fissures are found in the posterior midline, where they are often hidden under a sentinel pile. Fresh fissures look like an erosion. They are surrounded by normal anoderm, and at the base one can see delicate reddish muscle fibers. Chronic fissures have thickened, undermined margins. The whitish base, previously referred to as the pecten, is made up of transverse, fibrotic fibers of the internal sphincter muscle. Chronic fissures often terminate distally in a sentinel pile, while a polypoid mucosal swelling (hypertrophic papilla) is frequently found at the proximal apex. The fissure is tender to pressure and bleeds easily.

Therapy

Pain responds better to infiltration of the tissue underlying the fissure with a local anesthetic than to oral analgesics. This stops the pain and allows relaxation of the anal spasm. Fissures that are only a few weeks old can heal rapidly using this treatment. Freshening the margins of the fissure is helpful. Chronic fissures are excised under local anesthesia with scissors or with an electric knife. The excision is performed as a triangle with its base oriented distally to allow free drainage of secretions. The inflamed anoderm surrounding the fissure including the sentinel tag and the hypertrophic papilla is also excised (Figure 166). Lateral subcutaneous internal sphincterotomy under local anesthesia is recommended in cases with pronounced anal spasm. Postoperative treatment is with frequent baths, ointments, and regulation of bowel habits.

In cases with extensive tissue induration either surgical excision under anesthesia with or without a sphincterotomy, or manual anal dilatation (Lord's procedure [120]) is indicated.

Differential Diagnosis

An atypical, shallow, conspicuously indolent fissure with a poorly defined margin points toward a primary syphilitic chancre. The diagnosis is confirmed by the finding of Treponema pallidum in the dark-field examination of serous exudate from the ulceration. Serologic tests are frequently negative in the early course of the disease. Treatment is with systemic penicillin and local ointments. Broad-based, indolent ulcerations with a soft base and swollen edges, particularly in combination with fistulas, are typical in Crohn's disease. Treatment of the underlying disease is the main concern: The ulcerations should not be excised since wound healing is notoriously poor in florid Crohn's disease. Cold compresses and ointments are recommended instead (see Figures 172 and 372) [13, 25, 41, 47, 50, 128, 163, 222, 233, 234, 249, 279].

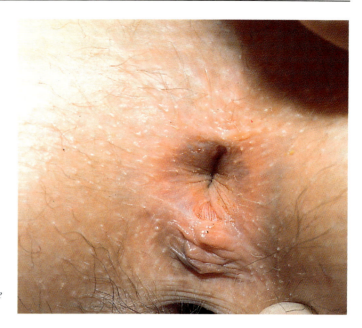

FIGURE 154
A red, 5 mm long, extremely tender acute fissure is seen in the anterior midline.

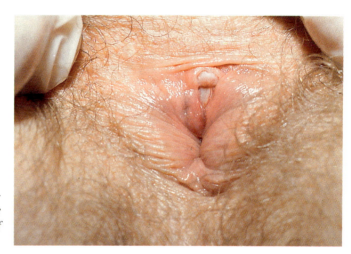

FIGURE 155
A chronic anal fissure is seen in the posterior midline after spreading the skin. The white base is formed by sclerotic fibers of the internal sphincter muscle.

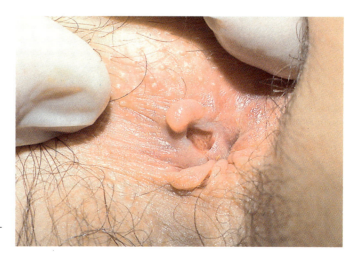

FIGURE 156
A fissure hidden under a sentinel pile is demonstrated by spreading the anal skin.

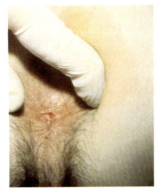
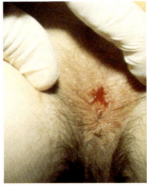

FIGURE 157
Left: acute fissure; right: the margins have been freshened by resecting transverse bands of scar tissue with scissors.

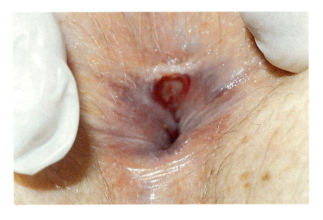

FIGURE 158
Chronic fissure with undermined edges and sclerotic muscle fibers of the internal sphincter at the base of the ulcer.

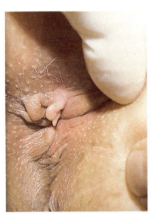
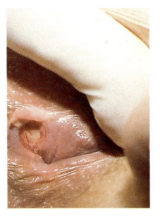

FIGURE 159
Sentinel pile in the posterior midline.

FIGURE 160
The fissure can be visualized by lifting the skin tag.

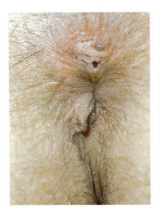
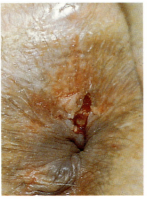

FIGURE 161
Fissure with the formation of pockets: A small round orifice like a fistula is seen in the posterior midline. Right picture: pocket is open, and the fissure is visible.

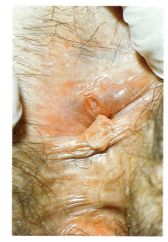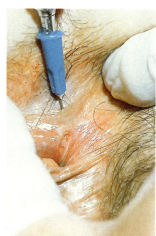

FIGURE 162
Injecting a local anesthetic under an acute fissure.

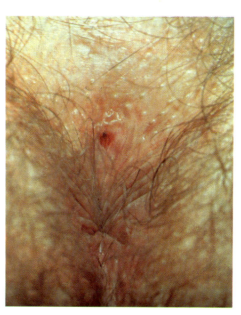

FIGURE 163
Microthrombosis in the posterior midline.

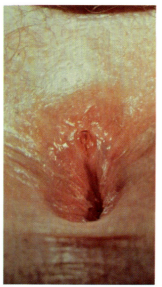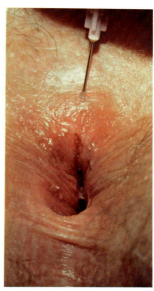

FIGURE 164
Three days later a fissure has developed at the site.

FIGURE 165
The fissure is healed by infiltration with a local anesthetic.

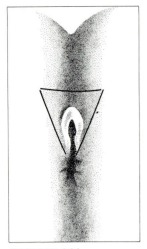 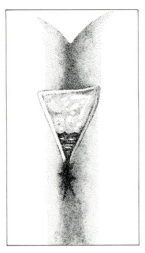

FIGURE 166
Triangular excision of the fissure with the base of the triangle outside to facilitate drainage. Skin tag and scar tissue are removed at the same time.

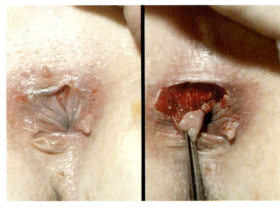

FIGURE 167
Left: fissure in the posterior midline bounded distally by a prominent undermined scar; right: the scar has been grasped with forceps and all scar tissue has been dissected off with an electric knife starting from a semicircular incision.

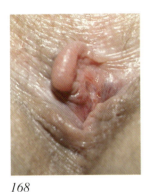 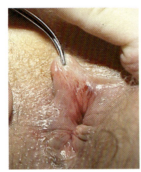 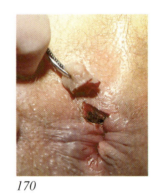 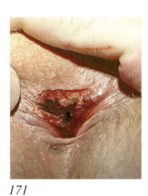

168 *169* *170* *171*

FIGURES 168–171
Skin tag and fissure are seen to the left of the posterior midline. In the midline there is a tear in the anoderm (fissure). The skin tag is palpated as a soft flap of skin. The fissure is very tender and bleeds easily when touched with a cotton swab. Under local anesthesia, the fissure can be visualized better by pulling the skin tag back with forceps. The skin tag is then resected with an electric knife, the fissure is removed with a triangular incision, and bleeding stopped with electrocautery.

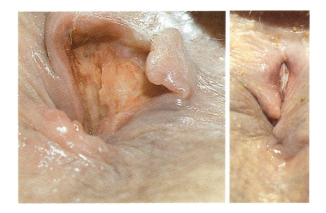

FIGURE 172
Ulcer in Crohn's disease: Unlike a fissure (right frame) it is shallow and indolent. The diagnosis is based on the demonstration of Crohn's disease in the gastrointestinal tract (see the chapter on anal and perianal alterations in Crohn's disease).

Anal Fistula (Fistula-in-ano)

Fistulas are caused by the penetration of pus from a suppurative focus, usually located in the anal glands in the crypts of Morgagni. If there is only a single opening, one refers to a sinus, or an incomplete or blind fistula. Fistulas can occur in actinomycosis, syphilis, gonorrhea, enteritis, Crohn's disease, and ulcerative colitis. Today tuberculosis is rarely a cause of fistulas.

Symptoms: Recurrent perianal swelling with tension pain and spontaneous discharge of pus and secretions. The orifice is frequently covered with skin and difficult to detect. It should be searched for immediately after material has been discharged. The fistulas often end beneath the mucosa, so that this must be penetrated with the probe to enter the crypts.

Therapy: The track of the fistula is probed with a cannula that is occluded with a stilette, which can be either sharp or blunt, as necessary.

A sharp stilette used for blind fistulas to penetrate into the crypt. When the tip of the cannula is in the anal canal, the stilette is removed and two lengths of monofilament nylon are inserted through the lumen and brought out through the anus. The cannula is then removed, and the nylon filaments are left in situ for drainage. After 2 to 3 weeks, all accessory tracts will have closed and secretion will cease. If the fistula is located submucously, subcutaneously, or intra-sphincteric, it can now be laid open with a cautery wire passed through the tract, or by cutting down with an inserted electric knife.

Transsphincteric fistulas and complex fistula systems must be treated surgically [25, 26, 41, 47, 50, 68, 129, 190, 222, 232, 235, 249, 253, 269, 279].

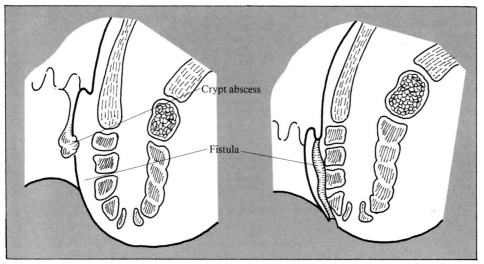

FIGURE 173

Steps in the development of a superficial fistula. Infection spreading from an inflamed crypt forms a fistula.

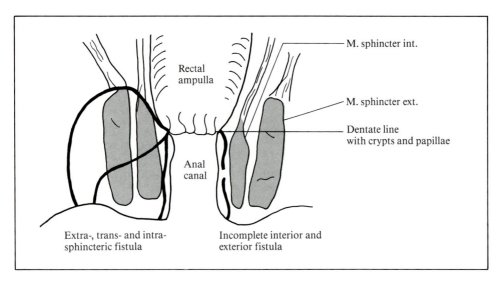

▲ **FIGURE 174**

Illustration of the main types of fistula. Extrasphincteric, transsphincteric, intrasphincteric, incomplete internal and external fistula. Pectinate line with crypts and papillae are also shown.

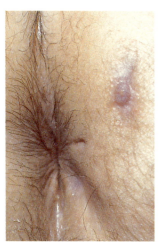 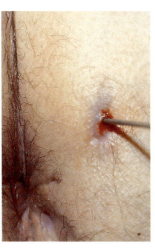

FIGURE 175

Sealed external fistula orifice in the right buttock. Right: Fistula is cannulated.

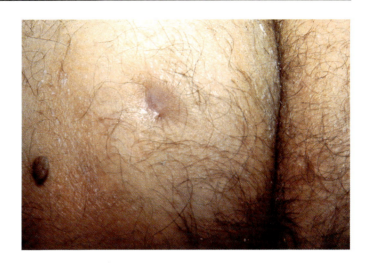

FIGURE 176
External fistula orifice in the left buttock covered by skin.

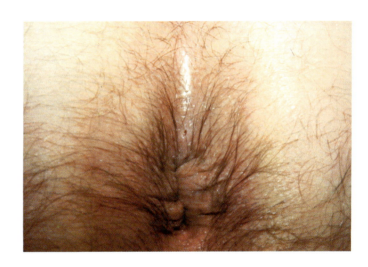

FIGURE 177
Fistula orifice in the posterior anal cleft.

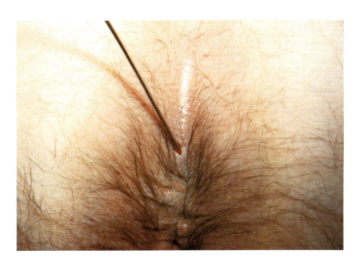

FIGURE 178
Probe in the fistula orifice (same patient as in Figure 177).

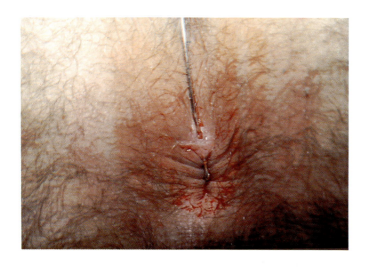

FIGURE 179
Blunt probe in an intrasphincteric fistula running subcutaneously and under the mucosa.

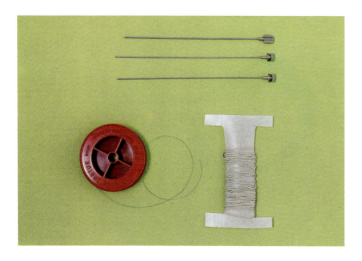

FIGURE 180
Instruments for treating fistulae (Breger). Above: cannula with both blunt and sharp pointed stilettes (the latter for perforating incomplete fistulas). Below: nylon filament and elastic.

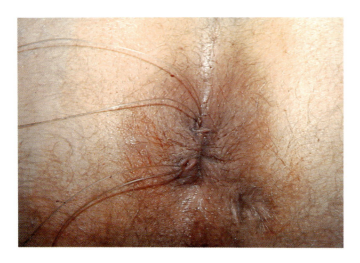

FIGURE 181
Fistula drained with doubled nylon filament.

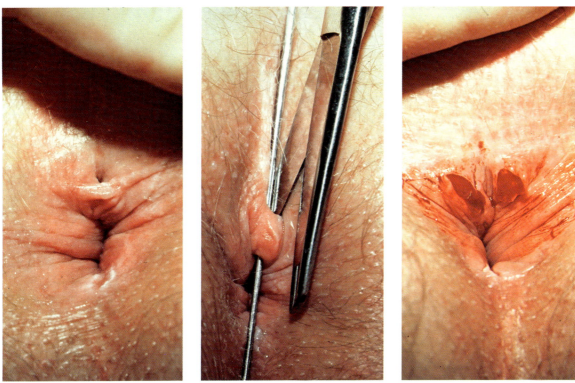

FIGURE 182–184
Fistula orifice in the posterior midline. The track of the intrasphincteric fistula is probed and then laid open with scissors.

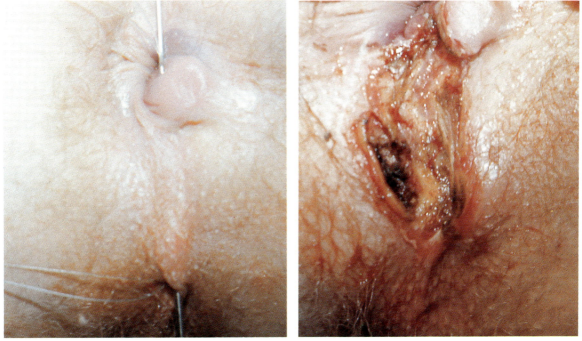

FIGURE 184a
The track of the intrasphincteric fistula is laid open with diathermy.

Anal Abscess

Incomplete internal fistulas arising in the crypts of Morgagni can lead to perianal abscesses. These cause severe pain, perianal swelling, and occasionally a raised temperature. A T-shaped or curved incision is made under superficial infiltration anesthesia, or freezing with ethyl chloride, and the wound is packed with gauze. Extensive abscesses must be drained under anesthesia [24, 25, 26, 41, 222, 234, 249].

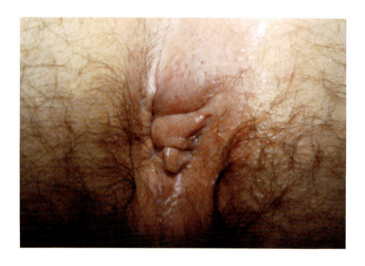

FIGURE 185
Slight bulging of the anoderm on the right caused by anal abscess.

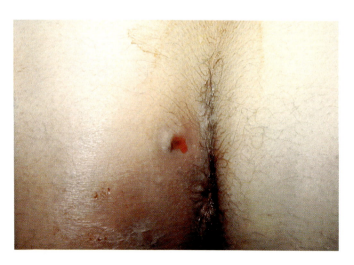

FIGURE 186
Induration of the left buttock with bleeding fistula orifice.

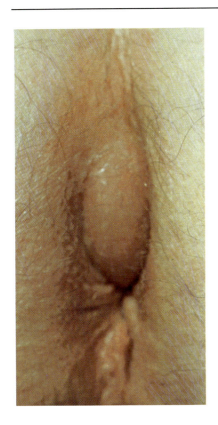

FIGURE 187
Tense and tender swelling in the posterior midline from a perianal abscess.

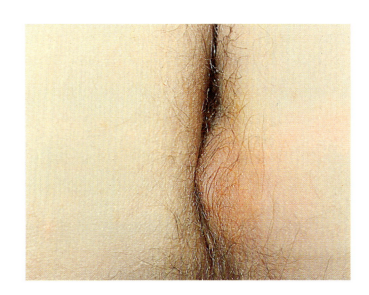

FIGURE 188
Perianal abscess on the right.

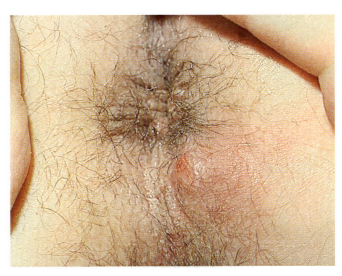

FIGURE 189
The bulging abscess is seen more clearly when the buttocks are spread.

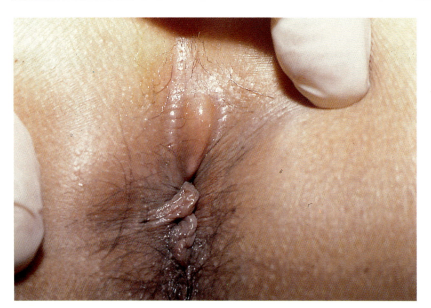

FIGURE 190

A swelling is seen on the right of the midline posteriorly. Digital examination reveals a firm, extremely tender mass.

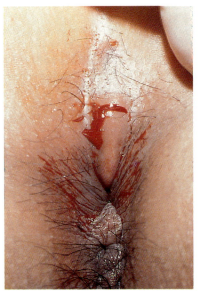

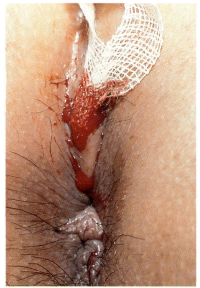

FIGURE 191

The same patient as in Figure 190. A curved incision is made under topical anesthesia. A substantial quantity of yellow pus is discharged.

FIGURE 192

The wound is packed with gauze for 2 to 4 days to aid drainage, and sitz baths and compresses are prescribed.

Further Disorders of the Anal Region

Anal Eczema

Anal eczema can either be acute or chronic. Erythema and weeping are the prominent features of acute eczema, while in the chronic form the skin is thickened, dry, and occasionally scaly. Pruritus and scratching are common features to both forms. Rhagades and bloody excoriations are frequent. The transition to normal anoderm can be either gradual or sharply demarcated.

Hemorrhoids play an important role in the etiology of anal eczema, although in many cases there are underlying causes such as contact allergy to toilet paper, drugs (hemorrhoid ointments and suppositories, laxatives, oral antibiotics and intestinal disinfectants, which disturb normal intestinal flora and suppress endogenous lactobacilli), traces of detergents in the underwear, soap, toiletries, and cosmetics. Candidiasis or oxyuriasis are sometimes responsible, while less common causes are prolapsed hemorrhoids or procidentia as well as prolonged diarrhea, especially in conjunction with colitis.

Therapy is determined by the etiology. Contact allergies are treated by avoiding the allergens that have been identified by sensitivity testing. Prolapsed hemorrhoids or rectal mucosa are treated by appropriate measures. Sclerosing internal hemorrhoids often has a beneficial effect, and topical corticosteroid ointments often bring rapid relief.

Bacterial superinfections must be treated with antibacterial ointments. Candida infections require specific antimycotic treatment, such as nystatin. Bran baths are beneficial when the skin is severely inflamed. Meticulous anal hygiene without the use of soap is essential [41, 160, 200, 222, 256, 257, 283].

Eczematous changes in the skin that have persisted for months or years and that are resistant to therapy must raise the suspicion of precancerous dermatoses such as Bowen's disease, or extramammary Paget's disease. Skin biopsies must be obtained for histological examination [200]. If the histology is positive, the affected area must be excised and the defect covered with a sliding flap. Another precancerous condition is lichen atrophicans, which causes kraurosis vulvae in postmenopausal women, and which is often accompanied by distressing pruritus. It causes a progressive involution and atrophy of the entire vulva and perineum. Inspection reveals chapped, parchment-like skin. Malignant changes must be ruled out by histology. Treatment consists of local and sometimes systemic estrogen therapy.

Psoriasis must be differentiated, although it only rarely presents as a solitary lesion in the perineum. The primary localization of psoriatic lesions are the elbows, the extensor surface of the knees, and the scalp, while the perianal region is afflicted only rarely. Typical of psoriasis are plaques that first appear as red areas, which are then rapidly covered with silvery or slightly opalescent scales; although these scales are frequently lacking on perianal lesions. Fine bleeding points are observed when the scales are scraped. The diagnosis of perianal psoriasis is greatly aided by the finding of concomitant lesions of other skin areas. Local treatment consists in the alternating application of topical corticosteroids and steroid-free keratolytics (or the carbol-fuchsin solution known as Castellani's paint) (see Figures 199–205).

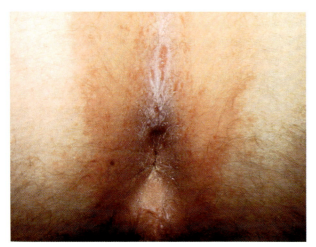

FIGURE 193
*Acute perianal eczema with rhagades and ex-
coriated skin.*

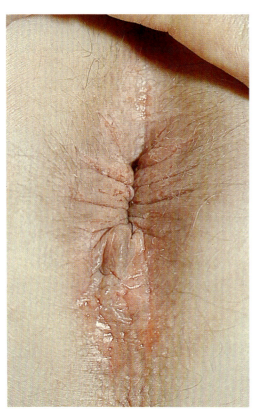

FIGURE 194
*Acute perianal eczema with rhagades and ex-
coriated skin.*

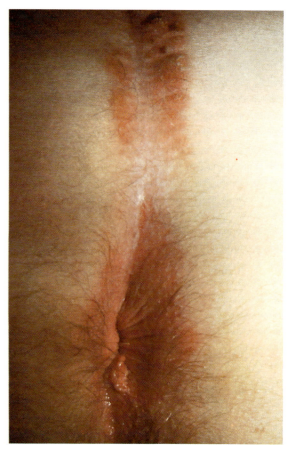

FIGURE 195
*Exacerbation of a chronic anal eczema with rha-
gades.*

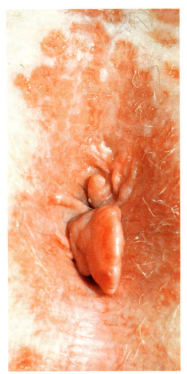

FIGURE 196
Skin tag with acute eczema.

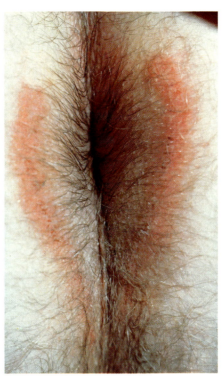

FIGURE 197
Eczema marginatum caused by infection with candida.

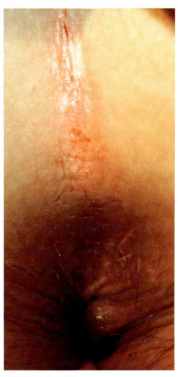

FIGURE 198
Weeping intertrigo in the anal cleft caused by excessive sweating.

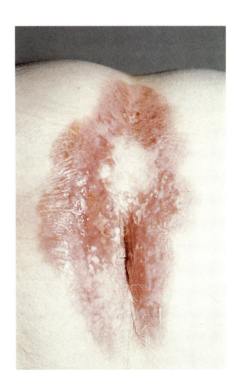

FIGURE 199
Paget's disease: This patient as well as those shown in Figures 200–205 had been treated for eczema for months without success.

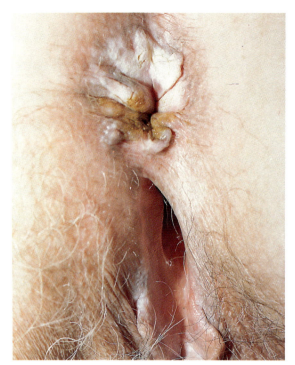

FIGURE 200
Kraurosis vulvae.

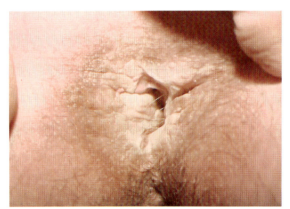

FIGURE 201
Perianal inflammatory infiltrations with rhagades seen in Crohn's disease.

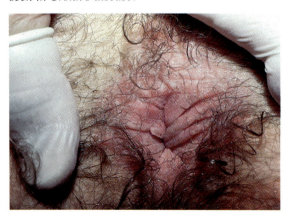

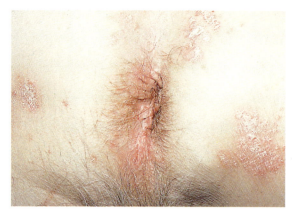

FIGURE 203
Perianal psoriasis.

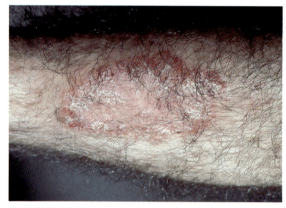

FIGURE 204
Psoriatic lesions on the forearm of the same patient.

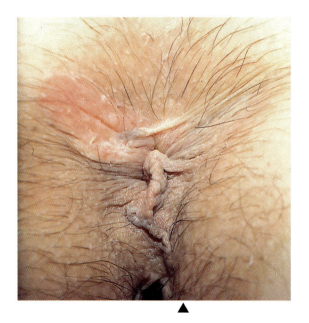

◀ FIGURE 202
Bowen's disease.

FIGURE 205
Basal cell carcinoma.

Pilonidal Sinuses (Sacral Dermoids)

Pilonidal sinuses are skin-lined cysts localized over the sacrum which are connected with the overlying skin by a narrow, epithelialized canal with an opening in the posterior midline. Secondary canals are seen occasionally. Infections of the cysts cause redness, swelling, and pain.

Pilonidal cysts are treated surgically by excision. If an abscess is present, it is drained first and the cyst is then removed 2 or 3 weeks later. In individual cases, a cure can be effected by curetting the cyst or by scrubbing with a fine brush.

A similar clinical picture is presented by the very rare perianal manifestation of hidradenitis

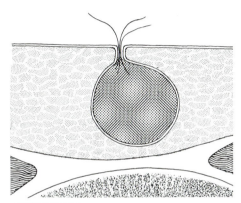

FIGURE 206
Pilonidal sinus.

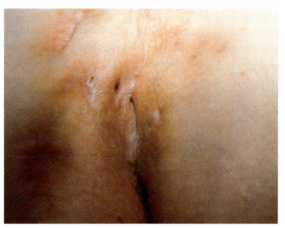

FIGURE 207
Numerous epithelialized orifices posterior to the anus leading to the pilonidal sinus over the sacrum.

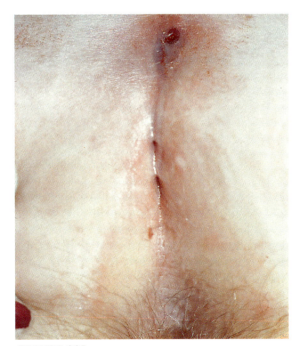

FIGURE 208
Scars overlying the sacrum with a fistula opening some distance from the anus found with a pilonidal sinus.

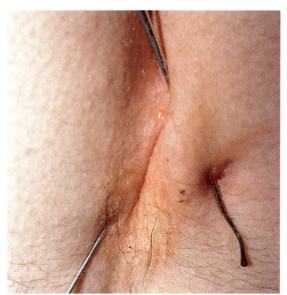

FIGURE 209
Pilonidal sinus. Fistulas are cannulated.

suppurativa, which causes invagination of the epidermis with infundibular scarring. Manifestation in other localizations such as the scrotum, inguinal region, the axilla, or retroauricular area are common. The therapy is surgical [41, 234, 249, 258, 271].

Proctalgia fugax (Anorectal Neuralgia, proctalgia nocturna)

This disorder is harmless but can be very annoying for the patient. The typical complaint are sudden episodes of deep-seated rectal pain, which can be lightening, spasmodic, or oppressive, and may be terminated by shifting position. The attacks usually occur during the early morning hours, thus awakening the patient. They are only short lived, lasting from a few seconds to about 15 minutes. They are occasionally accompanied by a false urge to defecate, nausea, retching, sweating, vertigo, or fainting. Proctalgia occurs twice as often in women between the ages of 30 and 50 as it does in men. Vascular spasms, frequently coincident with migraine, or spasms of the pelvic floor muscles are thought to be possible etiological factors. Differential diagnostic considerations must include coccygodynia, cauda equina syndrome, tabetic crisis, herpes simplex infection, anal fissures, acute thrombosed hemorrhoids, cryptitis, or abscesses, especially when the symptoms last for hours or longer. The diagnosis is based on the presenting complaints together with the normal findings of the proctological examination. Treatment of proctalgia fugax is usually unnecessary since the complaints only last a few seconds or minutes. They can be terminated by changing position, or by applying pressure to the perineum, inserting the finger into the rectum or by defecating. Often local heat application with hot-water bottles on the abdomen and perineum, or a warm bath rapidly alleviate the pain. Drugs such as spasmolytics or neuroleptics usually do not take effect until after the pain has gone away by itself, although nitroglycerine taken sublingually may be an exception. Sedatives taken in the evening may reduce the tendency toward attacks of proctalgia. On the other hand, operations in the perianal region such as sclerosant therapy or ligature of internal hemorrhoids can increase the predisposition for pain attacks [89, 168].

Pruritus ani

The anal region is the most common localization for pruritus. This is a subjective sensation caused by stimulation of finely branched, sensory nerves in the dermoepidermal boundary layer, eliciting the urge to scratch.

A slight burning sensation in the anal region is something everyone experiences occasionally. If the itching becomes more intense and occurs as annoying episodes, it can lead to the sensation of pain, which for the afflicted individual often takes on the dimensions of a true disease. It is no longer possible for the patient to differentiate between itching and pain, while the differences in the individual threshold intensity for both sensations adds to the difficulties. Slight irritation of the anal region is extremely unpleasant for sensitive patients, whereas others hardly seem to notice gross changes such as fissures or prolapse. Scratching provokes the synthesis and release of tissue mediators such as histamine, proteases, and prostaglandins. Small amounts of these can stimulate sensory receptors, which are numerous in the anal region. The stimulus is conveyed via peripheral nerves and the spinal cord to the central nervous system. The sensation can then trigger renewed scratching. Scratching also damages the epithelium, destroys the natural barrier against saprophytic bacteria, and paves the way for dermatitis. Pruritus usually subsides when the primary irritants are eliminated. During periods of strain or stressful situations, it can persist without a definite cause or histological alterations of the nerve ends. This can be seen, for example, after a bout of shingles.

The highly sensitive erogenic character, the anatomy, the funnel shape of the anus, the corrugated anoderm, and the vicinity to the intestine and vagina are all factors making the anal region a site of predilection for pruritus. Stool, sweat, and vaginal secretions can irritate the sensitive anoderm and cause itching. Stool particles retained in folds can macerate the skin and facilitate bacterial colonization. Liquid stools as in ulcerative colitis or Crohn's disease irritate the anal mucosa and the anal glands causing increased secretion. The same mechanism causes the hypersecretion observed in prolapsed mucosa or hemorrhoids, which leads to the irritation and inflammation of the anoderm also seen with vaginal discharge. Further causes are intestinal parasites, scabies, herpes genitalis, or a predisposition to elevated histamine concentrations in the skin as found in patients with atopic dermatitis. Also to be considered are tight-fitting trousers, underwear made from synthetic fabrics, or residual detergents in the underwear. Other factors are overheated rooms, prolonged sitting on plastic chairs, contact allergies against soaps, deodorants, ointments, colored toilet paper, or newsprint, or changes in the intestinal flora caused by antibiotics. One of the most common causes of anal itching is inadequate anal hygiene. Hot spices, coffee, chocolate and alcohol irritate the anal mucosa and are frequent causes of pruritus.

Careful inspection of the anal region and the anal canal is of decisive importance in the diagnostic work-up of patients with anal pruritus. It is easy to overlook subepidermal edema and minute superficial rhagades as signs of a dermatosis. An accurate history is just as important, since possible irritants can be identified by purposeful questioning. Important questions concern the consistency of the stool, the presence of mucoid or bloody discharge, anal hygiene habits, current medications, diabetes mellitus, and known contacts. A history of continence problems is a valuable indicator of a disturbed sphincter function, as are complaints of perianal moisture, soiled underwear, or prolapse. Anal itching that only occurs at night under warm bed-clothes is indicative of pinworm infestation. During the examination of the anal region, the buttocks must be widely spread so that every fold of the skin can be inspected. Stool particles in folds or under tags are easily missed but can be detected by wiping the perineum with cotton waste or fine paper. Bacteria and fungi are diagnosed in the stained or unstained smear or after culturing. Occasionally, the stool must be examined repeatedly to detect parasite eggs, pathogenic bacteria, and fungi. Vaginal discharge and kraurosis vulvae must be evaluated by a gynecologist. Digital examination of the anal canal might reveal a hypotonicity of the sphincter muscles, which would have an effect on continence, or hypertrophic anal papillae or tumors. Hemorrhoids, anusitis, cryptitis, and papillitis can be detected by anoscopy, which is performed as the next step. Proctoscopy should be carried out at every proctological examination so that inflammatory or neoplastic processes in the rectum will not be overlooked. After this, a general examination is performed to find diseases such as diabetes mellitus, leukemia, or Hodgkin's disease. Patch or scratch tests are done if an allergy is suspected.

Treatment of pruritus is easy if the underlying cause is known, which then has to be eliminated. Diseases such as tags, fissures, fistulas, prolapsed mucosa or hemorrhoids, intestinal parasites, vaginal discharge, diabetes mellitus, or diarrhea must be treated. Greatest attention must be directed toward anal hygiene: A constantly soiled anus defies all therapy. The anal region must be kept meticulously clean by washing or rinsing with lukewarm water. It should then be patted dry, not rubbed, with a soft cloth or soft paper tissues (for example, Kleenex). Sitz baths and compresses with chamomile have an antiphlogistic effect, while potassium permanganate and silver nitrate are useful astringents. Thin, absorbent, soft paper or muslin inserted in the underpants can help keep the anal region dry even during excessive perspiration. Tight-fitting trousers and underwear made of synthetic fibers should be avoided. All detergent residues must be rinsed from the underwear, since they can perpetuate eczemas. Short exposures to the sun or to ultraviolet light encourages healing.

Severe itching can be alleviated with corticosteroid ointments or by local steroid injections. If there is a superinfection with bacteria or fungi, the ointment must also contain antibiotics and antimycotics. The duration of steroid treatment must be limited, since it causes the skin to atrophy if applied over long periods of time. Antihistamines are only effective against urticaria. Treatment with protease inhibitors or inhibitors of prostaglandin synthesis may be of benefit.

Tranquilizers, sedatives, or physical exercise may helpful. Overweight patients with a funnel-shaped anus should be encouraged to lose weight. Neutral fat creams are good for dry perianal skin, common in elderly patients. Psychotherapy may be indicated in individual cases [25, 47, 93, 160, 168, 222, 249, 256].

Tumors of the Anal Region

Benign Tumors

The most common benign tumors of the distal anal canal are fibrous polyps (fibrotic hyperplasia of anal papillae), sentinel piles (polyps located distal to fissures), and condylomata acuminata (fibroepitheliomas). The diagnosis of these soft, villous tumors (condylomata acuminata) is made by histological examination of an excised nodule. Small pointed condylomata usually disappear rapidly after repeated swabbing with a 20% podophyllin solution or a 0.5% solution of podophyllotoxin in alcohol. The podophyllin solution must be rinsed off with water after 6 hours. Larger nodules are frozen with dry ice and scraped off. Various types of papilloma viruses (HPV) have been detected in the latter, and a viral etiology is considered very probable. Abscesses and perianal hematomas can resemble tumors. Bowen's disease in patients under the age of 40 is considered to be benign.

The most common benign tumors of the proximal anal canal are hyperplastic polyps, juvenile polyps (also known as retention polyps), tubulous, villous, or tubulo-villous adenomas. Hemangiomas, lipomas, and myomas are seen less frequently.

Rectal polyps can prolapse and resemble tumors of the anal canal.

Symptoms: A feeling of fullness, impaired anal hygiene, secretions, soiling of the underwear, and traces of blood on the toilet paper.

Diagnosis: Inspection of the anal region, palpation, and biopsy for histological examination.

Therapy: Resection of the tumors and histological examination [73, 74, 115, 162, 230, 235, 249].

Malignant Tumors

Squamous cell cancers, usually located in the distal portion of the anal canal, are the most common malignant tumors. Basaliomas, malignant melanomas, and Paget's disease are rare. Carcinomas in situ (Bowen's disease), and basaloid, plexiform, mucinous, mucoepidermoid, squamous, or anaplastic carcinomas arise in the epithelial transition zone of the proximal anal canal. Adenocarcinomas are the most common tumors at the anorectal junction. Mesenchymal tumors are very rare.

Leukoplacias with high-grade dysplasia are considered to be precancerous lesions.

Symptoms: A wide variety of complaints are seen depending on the localization and can be absent in the early stages of most tumors. Later, there is usually a dull, unrelenting pain in the anus, aggravated by defecation. Serosanguineous discharge is common.

Diagnosis: Inspection and digital palpation together with histological examination of biopsies.

Therapy: Treatment may be surgical and consist of amputation or wide local excision. Treatment with electrocoagulation or combined chemotherapy and radiation are less common. Squamous cell carcinomas are radiosensitive and are therefore amenable to x-ray contact therapy [3, 12, 21, 61, 73, 167, 186, 187, 188, 198, 200, 205, 207, 229, 240, 249, 282, 283].

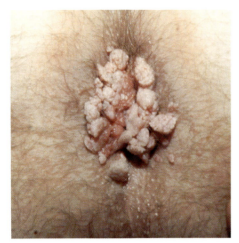

FIGURE 210
Condylomata acuminata.

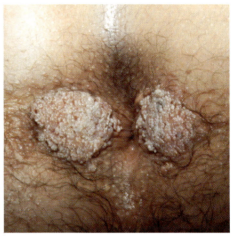

FIGURE 211
Condylomata acuminata; kissing lesions.

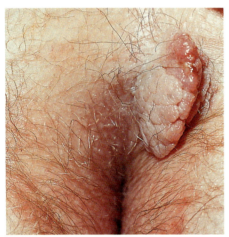

FIGURE 212
Condyloma acuminatum. Single sessile
lesion.

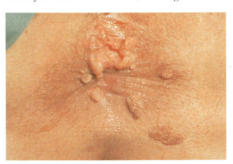

FIGURE 211a
Bowen's disease (cf. Figures 199, 202,
205). (Figures 211 and 213 were kindly
donated by Prof. Dr. med A. Akovbiantz,
Chief of the Surgical Clinic at the Waidspi-
tal, Zurich.)

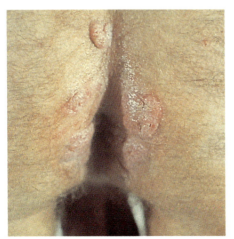

FIGURE 213
Condylomata lata (seropositive secondary
syphilis) (cf. 370, 371).

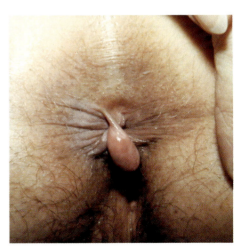

FIGURE 214
Pedunculated lipoma.

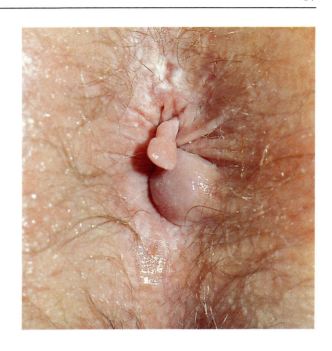

FIGURE 215
Perianal hematoma and fibroma.

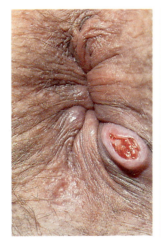 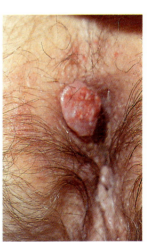

FIGURE 216
Spontaneously ruptured hematoma with skin tag on the left. Benign hyperkeratotic acanthoma on the right.

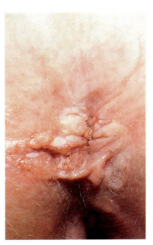 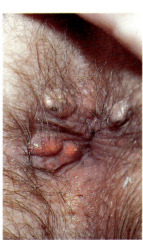

FIGURE 217
Acanthoma on the left, comedones on the right.

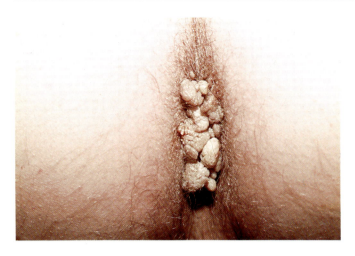

FIGURE 218
Condylomata acuminata. Multiple cauli-flower-like nodules cover the anus.

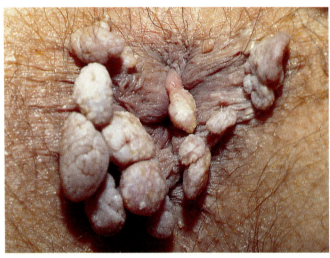

FIGURE 219
The individual nodules can be seen more readily after the buttocks have been spread. Some are pedunculated and arise from the perianal skin.

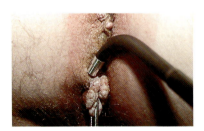 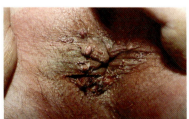 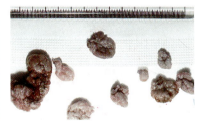

FIGURE 220
Left: The base of the large condyloma can be treated under local anesthesia by infrared coagulation. Center: The pedicle is then cut with scissors or diathermy with little bleeding. Right: Resected condylomata.

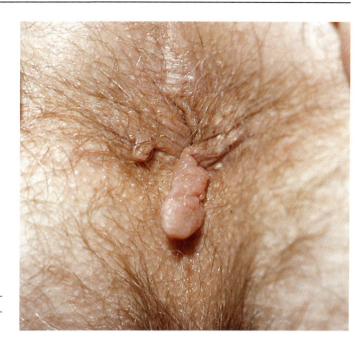

FIGURE 221
Perianal fibromas. Both are firm and painful when pinched, showing that they originate from sensitive skin.

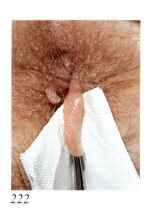

222

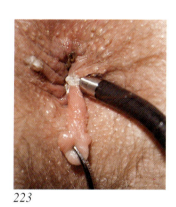

223

FIGURES 222–225
After local anesthesia the fibroma is grasped with forceps (Figure 222). The base coagulated with infrared coagulation (Figure 223). The base divided with scissors through coagulated tissue (Figure 224). Histologically, this was a fibroma (Figure 225).

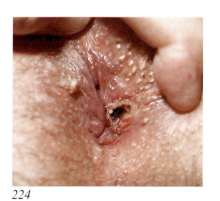

224

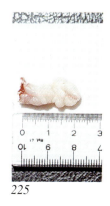

225

90

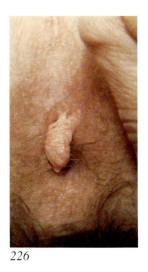

226

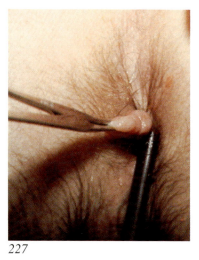

227

FIGURE 226–227.
Fibroma. Figure 227 shows it being
grasped with forceps and resected with an
electric snare.

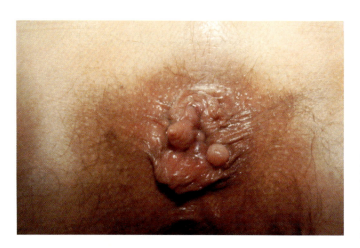

FIGURE 228
Tumors prolapsing through the anal canal.
To the left there is a prolapsed hypertrophic
anal papilla, below a prolapsed hemor-
rhoid, and at the right a prolapsed anal
polyp.

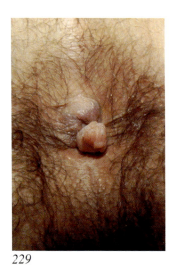

229

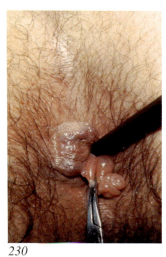

230

FIGURE 229–230
A hypertrophic anal papilla prolapsing
through the anal canal. In Figure 230, it has
been grasped with forceps and is being re-
sected with the electric snare.

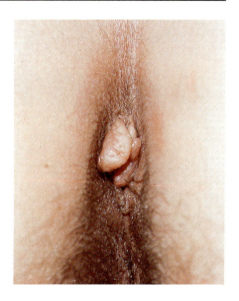

FIGURE 231
Sentinel piles.

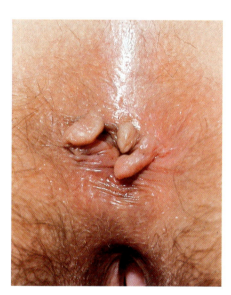

FIGURE 232
Three sentinel piles are easily seen after the buttocks are spread.
They hurt when pinched, which means they arise from sensitive
anoderm.

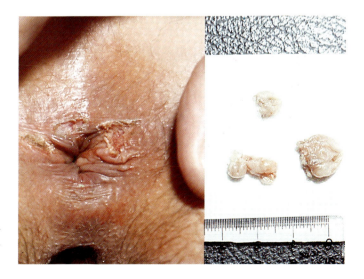

FIGURE 233
Same patient as above. The lumps are removed with diathermy under local anesthesia as they impeded anal hygiene.

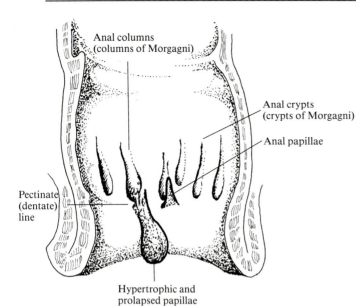

Anal columns
(columns of Morgagni)

Anal crypts
(crypts of Morgagni)

Anal papillae

Pectinate
(dentate)
line

Hypertrophic and
prolapsed papillae

FIGURE 234
Cross-section of the anal canal. The crypts of Morgagni with the anal papillae at their bases lie at the level of the pectinate line. A fibrotic hypertrophied papilla protrudes outside the anal canal.

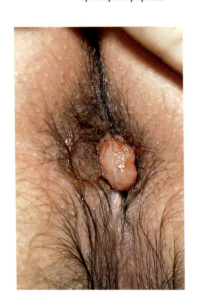

FIGURE 235
Prolapsed hypertrophied papilla. A smooth, whitish-yellow tumor appears in the anus. The tumor can be pushed back into the anal canal and its pedicle felt there during digital examination.

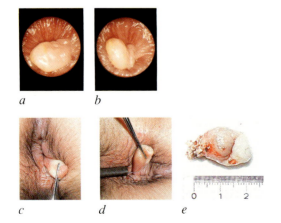

a   *b*

c   *d*   *e*

FIGURE 236 (a–e)
Endoscopic view of the hypertrophied papilla seen in Figure 235 (a + b). Removal of the tumor under local anesthesia. Local anesthesia is necessary since the tumor is an appendage of the sensitive anoderm. The tumor is grasped with forceps and elevated (c). The electric snare is then looped around it (d) and it is resected (e).

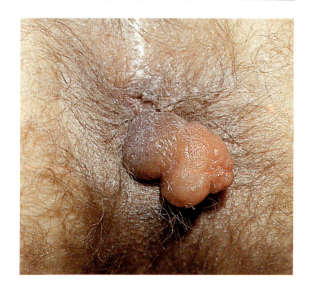

FIGURE 237
Partial mucosal prolapse. A smooth red lump is seen on the right. It is based on the reddish-blue mucosa of the anal canal which also protrudes slightly. It can be replaced manually.

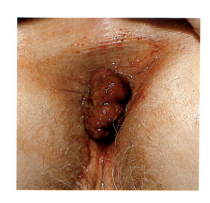

FIGURE 238
Prolapsed adenoma. A finely lobulated tumor that bleeds easily is situated in the anal orifice.

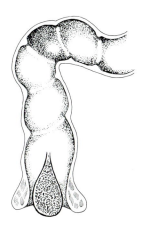

FIGURE 240–241
This tumor could not be replaced into the rectum. Digital examination revealed a peduncle. The electric snare was passed around this, and the tumor resected at its base. Endoscopy showed the resection site to be just proximal to the anal canal.

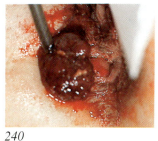

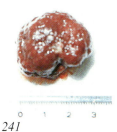

FIGURE 239
Schematic drawing of a prolapsed pedunculated rectum tumor. The histological diagnosis was a papillomatous rectal adenoma (Institute of Pathology, University of Bern).

240

241

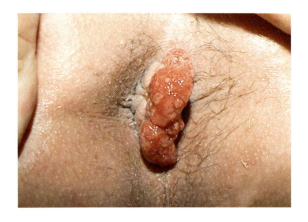

FIGURE 242
Prolapsed tubulovillous adenoma. This is a soft tumorous mass which can be pushed back into the anal canal.

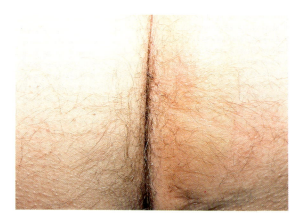

FIGURE 243
The adenoma can be returned to the rectum. Its base is felt above the anal canal.

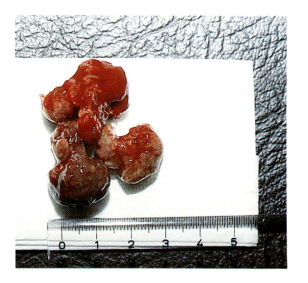

FIGURE 244
Endoscopy showed that the tumor masses originated just above the anal canal on the left side. The electric snare was passed around the base, and the tumor resected. The histological diagnosis was a tubulovillous adenoma (Institute of Pathology, University of Bern).

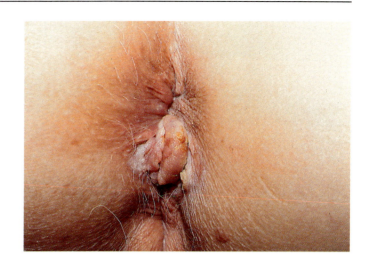

FIGURE 245
Bowenoide precarcinoma.

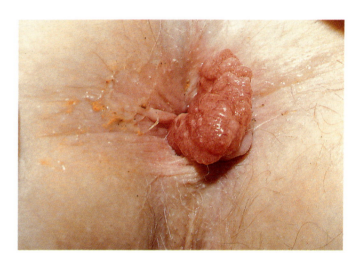

FIGURE 246
Prolapsing rectal carcinoma.

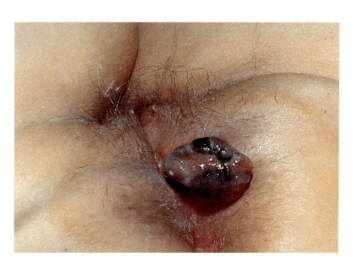

FIGURE 247
Malignant melanoma.

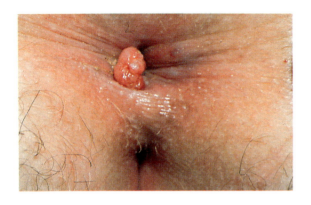

FIGURE 248
Adenocarcinoma. Palpation revealed a granular, hard infiltration in the anal canal.

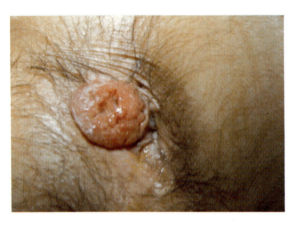

FIGURE 249
Squamous cell carcinoma.

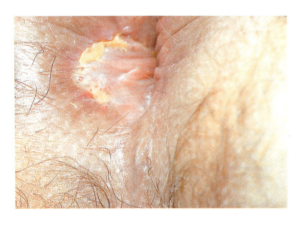

FIGURE 249 A
The same patient as in Figure 249. The tumor was treated with 3000 r (contact irradiation).

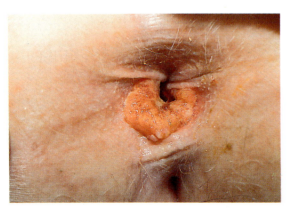

FIGURE 250
Anal carcinoma.

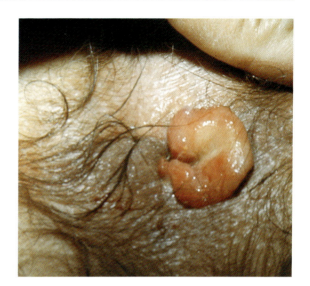

FIGURE 251

Mixed tumor: squamous cell-adenocarcinoma presenting as a hard, immobile, reddish lump at the anal verge. Digital examination of the anal canal revealed firm induration deep to the visible lump.

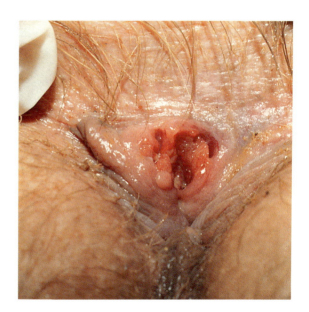

FIGURE 252

Granular tumor masses are seen in the anal canal. Histological examination of biopsy material results in the diagnosis of a squamous cell-adenocarcinoma (Institute of Pathology, University of Bern). Therapy: proctectomy.

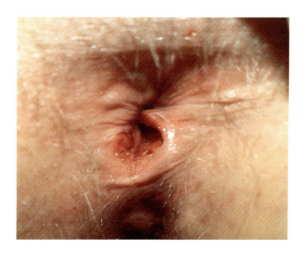

FIGURE 253

Cloacogenic carcinoma. An ulcer with a granular base is seen in the anterior midline. The base of the ulcer is hard and tender to touch (Institute of Pathology, University of Bern). Therapy: proctectomy.

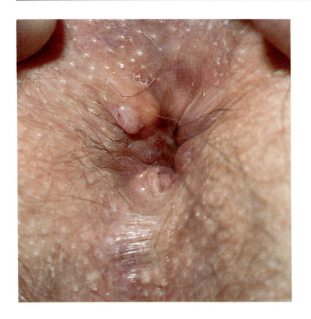

FIGURE 254
Mucinous carcinoma. There is a white nodule on the ridge seen on the left of the posterior midline at 10 o'clock. There is a fistula opening on the apex of the nodule which can be followed into the anal canal with a blunt probe. The tissue is infiltrated and hard. The infiltration extends to the anal canal. Histological examination of biopsied material reveals a mucinous carcinoma (Institute of Pathology, University of Bern). Therapy: proctectomy.

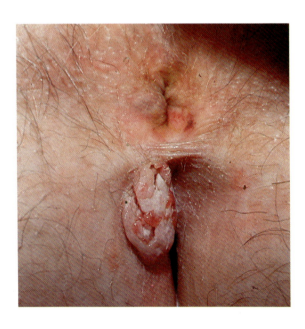

FIGURE 255
Epidermoid carcinoma. An ulcerated, bleeding, granular tumor is seen on the perineum near the vagina. The tumor is not tender, and has a slightly firm consistency. Microscopical examination of tissue removed from the center of the tumor revealed an incipient epidermoid carcinoma (Institute of Pathology, University of Bern). Therapy: local excision.

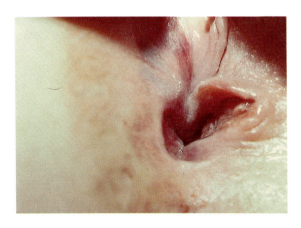

FIGURE 256
Ulcerated epidermoid carcinoma. Therapy: proctectomy.

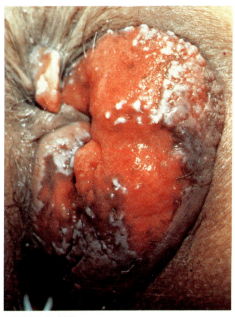

FIGURE 257
Extensive ulcer with a firm consistency to the right of the anus. The patient had thought she was suffering from hemorrhoids for more than 6 months. Microscopic examination revealed a squamous cell carcinoma. (Pathological Institute of the University of Bern).

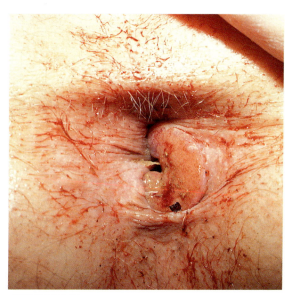

FIGURE 258
Squamous cell carcinoma

FIGURE 259 ➤
Prolapsing adenocarcinoma. A dusky-red, finely lobulated tumor is located in the anus. It is firm to the touch and cannot be replaced into the rectum. Its origin can be palpated directly above the anal canal.

FIGURE 260 ➤➤
The tumor was resected at its base with the electric snare and sent in for histological examination. This revealed an adenocarcinoma of the rectum (Institute of Pathology, University of Bern).

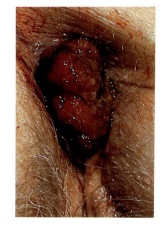 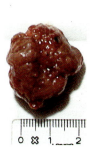

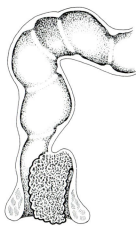

FIGURE 261
Schematic drawing of the rectal tumor protruding into the anal canal.

Prolapse

One must differentiate between mucosal prolapse, in which only the mucosa protrudes through the anus, and rectal prolapse, which affects all layers of the rectum wall. Rectal prolapse is divided into four stages: invagination not visible from the outside; visible prolapse returning spontaneously; visible prolapse requiring manual reduction; and the final stage, in which the rectum never returns to the normal position. At the beginning, the prolapse only appears during heavy straining, but later it occurs at every defecation or even while standing or walking. The prolapse causes bleeding, mucous discharge, and is frequently associated with stool incontinence.

A prolapsed mucosa has radial folds and feels thin when grasped between the thumb and index finger. Prolapsing hemorrhoids or rectal polyps are contributory factors in the pathogenesis of mucosal prolapse.

Minor mucosal prolapse is treated by reattaching the mucosa to the wall of the rectum by means of sclerosant therapy or rubber band ligature [13, 25, 131, 155, 175, 235].

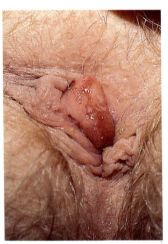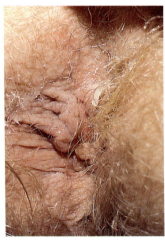

FIGURE 262
Partially prolapsed mucosa, before and after reduction.

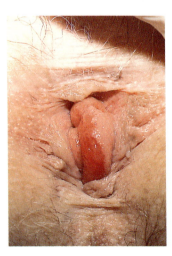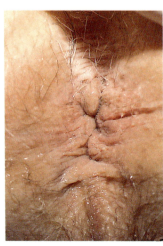

FIGURE 263
A similar case.

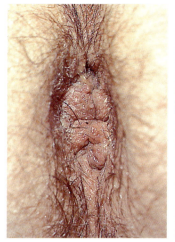
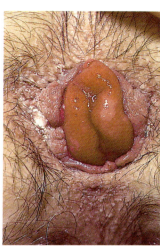

FIGURE 264
Bilateral mucosa prolapse. The mucosa is edematous, thick, and red. There is mucus discharge.

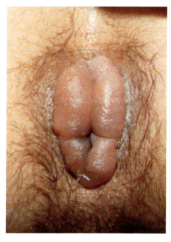
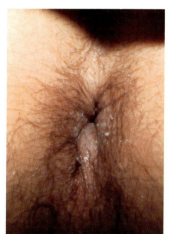

FIGURE 265
Acute, circular mucosal prolapse with pale red edema, and after manual reduction.

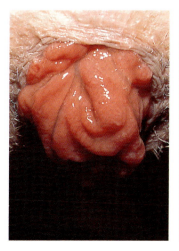
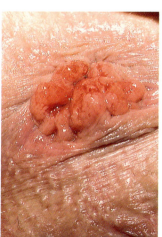

FIGURE 266
Circular mucosal prolapse with radial folds in the mucosa, reduced manually on the right.

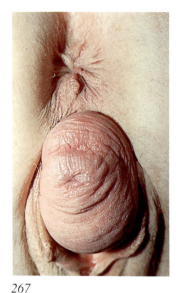
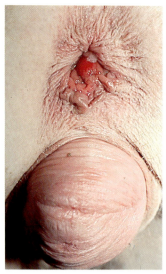

FIGURE 267
Cervical prolapse in procedentia.

FIGURE 268
During straining there is also a partial mucosal prolapse in the anterior midline.

267   268

Incarcerated Prolapse

This term refers to a hitherto reversible prolapse that swells acutely at the end of a defecation and is then no longer reducible. Within minutes, the circulation in the prolapsed structures is compromised by a spasm of the sphincter muscle. The mucosa swells grossly, and edema develops in the course of several hours. Inspection reveals tense, purple lumps surrounded by bright red edematous mucosa.

Therapy: Reposition should only be attempted when the surrounding edema is still soft and pliable. The edema can be decreased by the application of a corticosteroid ointment. The prolapse is then generously coated with lubricant or the steroid ointment and carefully reduced by applying gradually increasing pressure. It is not recommended to anesthetize the sphincter, since the sphincter tension is necessary to prevent recurrent prolapse. The patient must remain in a prone position for at least 15 minutes following the successful reposition. It is advisable to apply a compression bandage before the patient leaves the office. A mild laxative is prescribed to regulate the bowels.

No attempt should be made to reduce a prolapse that has lasted for several hours, is hard from edema, and has taken on a bluish-black discoloration. Treatment consists of bed rest, preferably in the prone position, cold compresses, laxatives to achieve liquid stools, and administration of analgesics and, if necessary, antiinflammatory drugs.

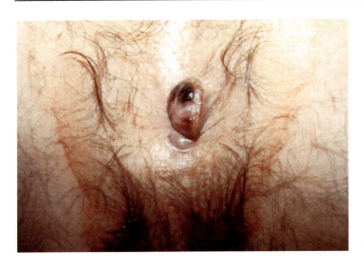

FIGURE 269
Incarcerated prolapsed mucosa with a thrombosed hemorrhoid.

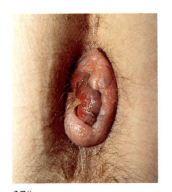 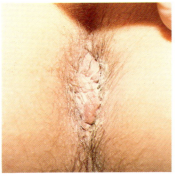

270   271

FIGURES 270–271
Prolapsed and incarcerated piles. The edematous perianal skin bulges outwards around the entire circumference of the anus. In the center a dark-red pile is visible. After applying a lubricant the pile was slowly forced back into the anal canal with a finger.

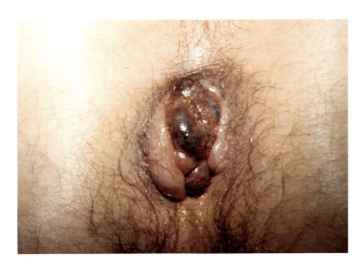

FIGURE 272
Incarcerated prolapsed mucosa with extensive thromboses and edematous swelling of surrounding tissue.

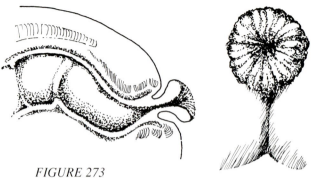

FIGURE 273
Schematic diagram of a mucosal prolapse.

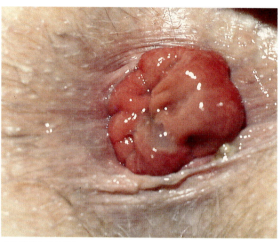

FIGURE 274
Circular mucosal prolapse with radial folds in the mucosa.

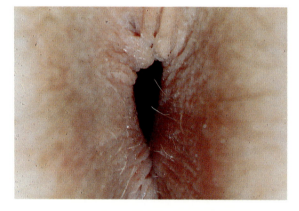

FIGURE 275
After reduction of circular mucosal prolapse. A gaping anal canal is found on inspection.

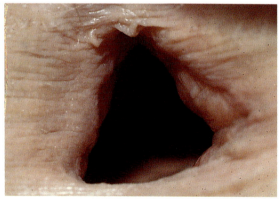

FIGURE 276
Spreading the buttocks causes the anal canal to open widely.

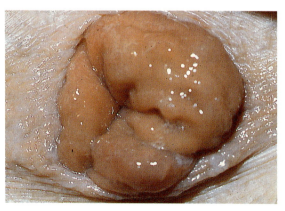

FIGURE 277
Pink mucosa, with radial folds appears at straining.

Total Circular Prolapse

With total circular prolapse, all layers of the intestinal wall come out through the anus.

Symptoms: Sensation of fullness, mucous or bloody discharge, incontinence [175, 221].

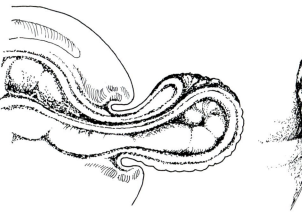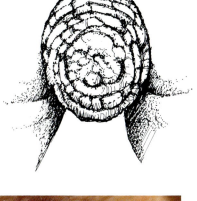

FIGURE 278
Schematic drawing illustrating the protrusion of all layers of the intestinal wall, which is in effect a hernia of the pelvic floor. The typical circular mucosal folds are shown.

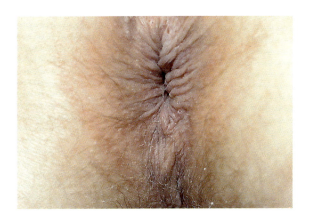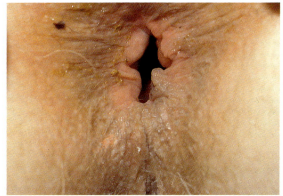

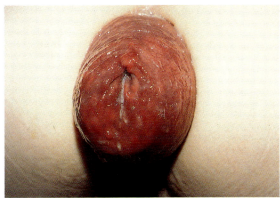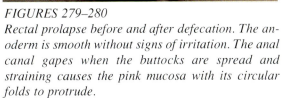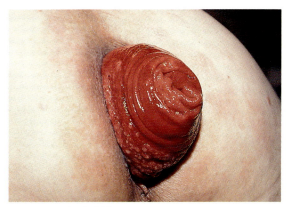

FIGURES 279–280
Rectal prolapse before and after defecation. The anoderm is smooth without signs of irritation. The anal canal gapes when the buttocks are spread and straining causes the pink mucosa with its circular folds to protrude.

FIGURES 281–282
Figure 282 shows the prolapse after defecation. The rectum extends like a telescope for almost 10 cm outside the anus and has the typical circular folds.

Diseases of the Rectum

Melanosis coli

The intestinal mucosa exhibits reticular or macular deposits of lipofuscin, which is found both in histiocytes as well as extracellularly. The condition is reversible. It occurs after prolonged use of laxatives containing senna leaf, aloe, or rhubarb. The proctoscopic findings are impressive but without clinical relevance [41, 203, 237, 249].

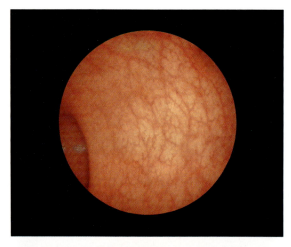

FIGURE 283
Endoscopic view of normal reddish mucosa with its vascular network easily visible, and its smooth, shiny surface.

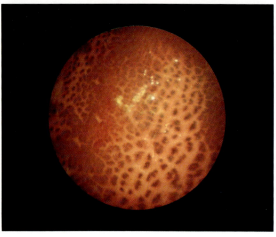

FIGURE 284
Macular pigmentation of the rectal mucosa in melanosis coli.

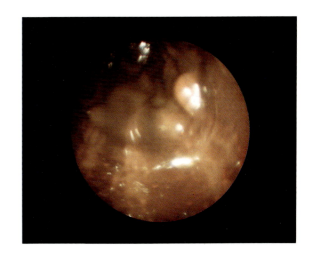

FIGURE 285
Melanosis with a pea-sized mucosal polyp.

Internal Mucosal Prolapse, Solitary Ulcer

A circumscribed area of inflammation is found on the ventral surface of the rectum. It is caused by a prolapse of the anterior wall of the rectum during straining. An ulcer often develops from the constantly recurring mechanical irritation. The ulcer has a bizarre shape, is oval or round, and has a yellowish or white fibrinous base. Characteristic for the histology is a fibromuscular obliteration of the lamina propria. The treatment consists of preventing excessive straining with bulk laxatives or lubricants. The endoscopic changes take months or years to disappear.

In individual cases, the mucosa can be prevented from prolapsing by gathering and fastening it with a rubber-band ligation. Transabdominal proctopexy can cure resistant ulcers. According to Madigan and Morson, however, any treatment is unsuccessful [41, 57, 123, 141, 154, 192, 217, 218, 238, 244].

FIGURE 286
Prolapse proctitis: A band of red and edematous mucosa is seen anteriorly which prolapses into the endoscope during straining.

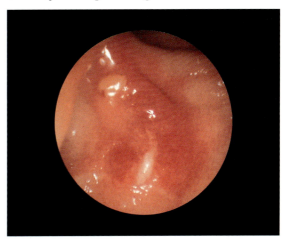

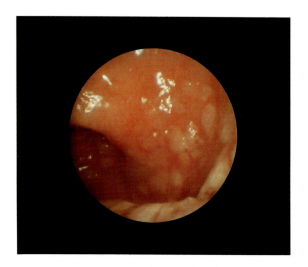

FIGURE 287
Inflammation from prolapse with thickened granular mucosa.

FIGURE 289
Multiple ulcers.   ▼

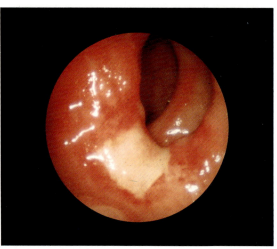

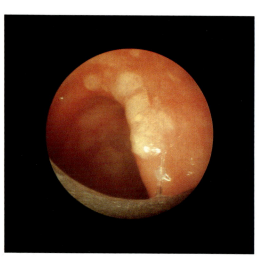

FIGURE 288
Solitary ulcer with whitish base surrounded by edematous mucosa.

FIGURE 290 (a + b)
Marginal bleeding solitary ulcer (a). Shallow ulcer with reddened edematous mucosa surrounding it (b).   ▼

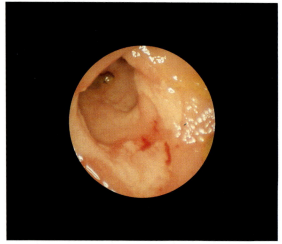

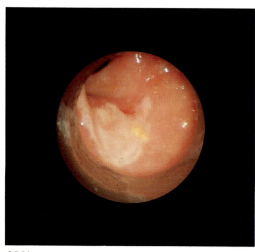

290a

290b

Inflammatory Diseases of the Rectum

A distinction is made between nonspecific inflammatory disorders such as ulcerative colitis and Crohn's disease, and specific inflammation caused by radiation, bacteria, viruses, antibiotics, and parasites. Bloody diarrhea is the main symptom. Endoscopic examination shows mucosal edema, erosions, aphthous ulcers, fibrinous membranes as well as small or large areas of necrosis [80, 81, 105].

The various forms cannot be differentiated visually. The diagnosis is based on the history, clinical presentation, mucosal biopsy with histological examination [97], and laboratory results [82]. Ulcerative colitis and Crohn's disease have become more common in recent years, as have sexually transmitted anorectal diseases. Less common are cases of proctitis caused by radiation, bacteria, or parasites.

Nonspecific Inflammation of the Rectum

Ulcerative Colitis (Idiopathic Ulcerative Colitis)

Ulcerative colitis is a chronic noninfectious inflammation of the mucosa of the rectum and colon with repeated remissions and exacerbations causing mucosal bleeding and ulceration. It most frequently affects young adults with an equal distribution between males and females.

Etiology: unknown. A number of findings seem to indicate that immunological reactions are an important factor in the occurrence and chronic course of the disease. The patients are usually emotionally disturbed with a disposition toward depression and introversion.

Symptoms: Bloody, purulent, and mucous diarrhea is the main symptom in the typical form.

Diagnosis: Endoscopy reveals an edematous, velvety, dark-red mucosa coated with mucus. Minimal trauma causes pinpoint bleeding. Ulcers are rarely seen in the rectum, which is why the term *hemorrhagic proctitis* is more fitting. The disease tends to spread proximally. The proximal boundary with healthy mucosa is often sharply demarcated. Microscopic examination of biopsy material can aid in the diagnosis. The most gentle biopsy method is with the suction biopsy instrument developed by Heinkel [97]. Acute salmonellosis and bacillary dysentery can be ruled out by bacteriological examination of the stool and the absence of specific antibodies in the blood.

Therapy consists of the oral administration of sulfasalazine or 5-aminosalicylic acid, in combination with corticosteroids in severe cases. When the disease is restricted to the rectum, the rectal application of these drugs as suppositories or enemas is preferred, although supplementary oral treatment is always possible. Sulfasalazine is split by the intestinal flora to yield the carrier substance sulfapyridine and the therapeutic substance 5-aminosalicylic acid (mesalazine). The majority of the adverse effects of sulfasalazine (nausea, vomiting, thrombocytopenia, agranulocytosis, hemolytic anemia, lupus erythematosus-like symptoms, and disturbances of male fertility) can be attributed to the carrier substance sulfapyridine. Preparations containing only mesalazine are better tolerated. Special preparations release the drug in the terminal ileum, so that it is available for local effect on the inflamed mucosa in the colon. In the acute phase, 3–4 g of sulfasalazine is given daily divided into 3 or 4 doses. For maintenance therapy, 1.5–2 g are considered adequate. A blood count must be taken every 2 months. The equipotent dose of mesalazine 5-ASA is 1.5–3 g for acute disease, and 0.75–1.5 g to prevent relapses. This drug is recommended for young men since it does not affect fertility [69]. Adverse effects can occur if salicylates are not tolerated. Corticosteroids are ineffective in preventing recurrences [6, 30, 46, 63, 87, 142, 179, 242, 249].

Complications: General complications are less common in ulcerative colitis than in Crohn's disease (see below). On the other hand, the risk of developing colon cancer increases with the duration of the disease.

Total proctocolectomy is indicated in cases of malignant degeneration, impending toxic megacolon, or intractable cases with severe impairment of general health [83, 176, 179, 226].

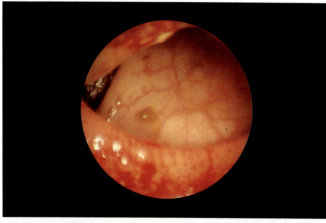

FIGURE 291
Proctitis of the distal rectum: Red mucosa which bleeds easily is seen in the foreground while normal mucosa with its vascular network is visible behind it.

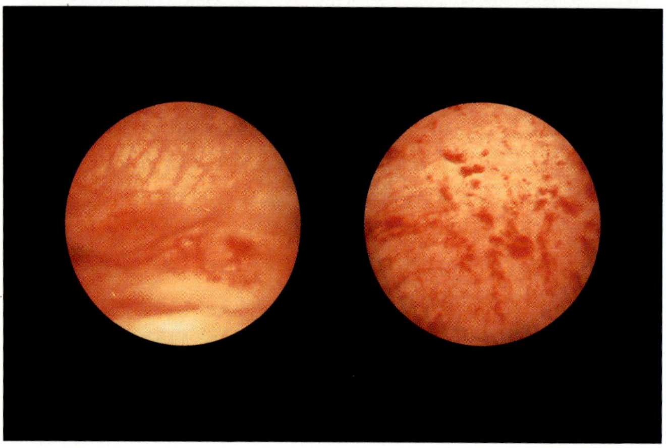

FIGURE 292
Hemorrhagic proctitis.

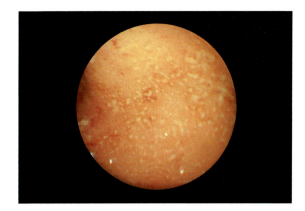

FIGURE 293
Ulcerative colitis.

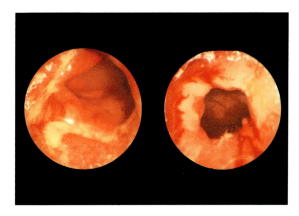

FIGURE 294
Ulcerative colitis (purulent type).

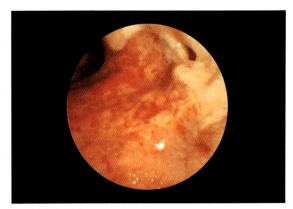

FIGURE 295.
Full-blown picture of ulcerative colitis with bloody,
purulent mucosa.

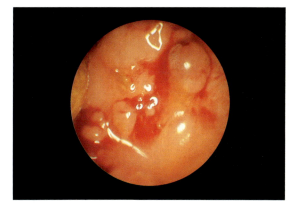

FIGURE 296
Ulcerative colitis with pseudopolyps.

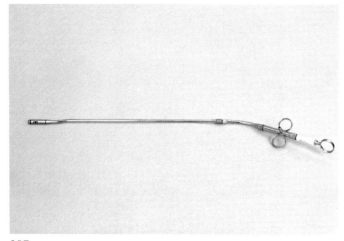

297

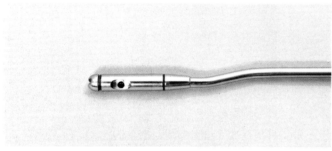

298

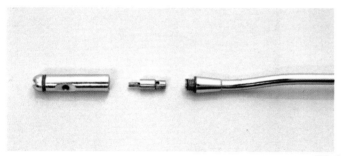

299

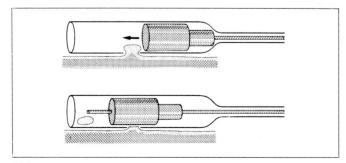

300

FIGURES 297–300
Instrument for obtaining suction biopsies of the mucosa as described by Heinkel [97]. The mucosa is sucked through a 2 mm side-hole and cut off with a sliding barrel.

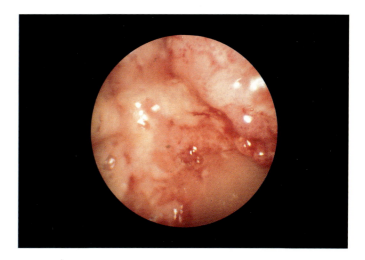

FIGURE 301
Ulcerative colitis with pseudopolyps.

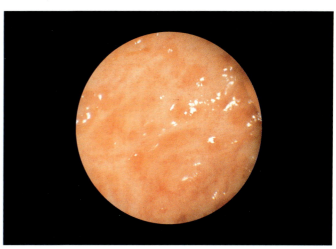

FIGURE 302
Ulcerative colitis in the process of healing
with mucosal scarring and pseudopolyps.

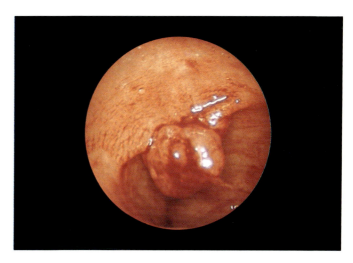

FIGURE 303
Carcinoma in a patient with ulcerative
colitis of 10 years standing.

Regional Colitis (Granulomatous Colitis, Ileitis, Crohn's Disease)

In regional colitis, not only the mucosa is affected as in ulcerative colitis, but also deeper layers of the wall including the serosa. This often leads to the development of fissures, fistulas, and stenoses. The localization is usually circumscribed and patchy with predominant involvement of the ileum and the colon, although the rectum is often spared. The circumscribed lesions are characteristically sharply demarcated and separated by regions of normal mucosa [37, 38, 63, 98, 179].

Symptoms: Diarrhea, pain, bouts of fever, extraintestinal inflammatory reactions, and partial intestinal obstruction. Bleeding is rare. Anal changes such as ulcers and fistulas are common. The latter are frequently the first symptom, which is why an atypical anal fistula should always raise the suspicion of regional enteritis. The fistulas can give rise to perianal abscesses or penetrate into the gut, the bladder or the vagina.

Findings: Endoscopy reveals a red, thick, edematous mucosa without visible vessels. Fine tears in the mucosa and deep longitudinal ulcers are frequently observed.

In about 20–30% of the cases, histological examination of biopsy material reveals the typical epithelioid granulomas of Crohn's disease [82, 238].

Radiological examinations demonstrate the reduced distensibility of the affected gut. The lumen is frequently narrowed to the thickness of a pencil and is eccentric or funnel-shaped. The mucosa has a cobblestone appearance, with spicules located between the cobblestones.

Treatment is with sulfasalazine or mesalazine with or without cortisone as in ulcerative colitis (see above), elemental diet or total parenteral nutrition.

General complications of regional enteritis are erythema nodosum, arthritis, uveitis, toxic megacolon (although the latter is not as common as in ulcerative colitis), and anal fistulas. In long-standing disease there is also the danger of malignant degeneration [37, 38, 66].

Anal and Perianal Changes in Regional Colitis (Crohn's Disease)

In regional colitis, all layers of the intestinal wall including the serosa are affected. This is the reason for the common occurrence of fissures, fistulas and stenoses, which can be an early symptom of Crohn's disease. The main cause is the loose stool, which irritates the anal mucosa and the perianal skin leading to local inflammation. Inflammatory, ulcerating processes in the rectal mucosa can also spread to surrounding structures causing abscesses and fistulas. The irritated, inflamed perianal skin is macerated with erosions and tiny tears, which are colonized by bacteria and fungi. The results are rhagades and inflammatory infiltration. Pre-existent skin tags become edematous and swollen.

The retention of stool in folds of the anoderm cause local inflammation: The tissue loses its elasticity and can tear during the passage of a stool. Chronic inflammation and superinfection further the development of ulcers. The ulcers in regional enteritis do not have the punched-out appearance found in fissures; the edges are edematous, thickened, and frequently undermined. They are also not situated in the midline and are not tender to touch like a fissure. The surrounding skin has a bluish hue. The inflammatory tissue reactions can affect the sphincter causing incontinence or, more commonly, narrowing of the anal canal as a result of fibrosis. In digital examination the anal canal is found to be indurated and scarred, and frequently cannot be entered with the endoscope. Since the stenosis is no obstacle for the thin stools, it rarely causes symptoms. Involvement of the anal crypts caused by the continual irritation can lead to cryptitis and to abscesses in the crypts. The latter can progress to form fistulas. Complex fistula tracts with multiple openings are not uncommon in patients with regional enteritis. Typical for the fistulas of Crohn's disease are the paucity of symptoms, the chronicity, and the induration of the fistula tracts with livid coloring of the surrounding skin. In every case of atypical anal disease, one should keep in mind the possibility of regional enteritis and search for typical signs in the rest of the digestive tract.

The therapy of perianal and anal manifestations of regional colitis is primarily conservative and demands a great deal of patience from both the physician and the patient. The mainstay of therapy is the treatment with sulfasalazine, mesalazine 5-aminosalicylic acid, steroids, or metronidazole. Anal hygiene is important, and the anus should be cleansed with water after every defecation. A perpetually soiled anus thwarts the success of the otherwise effective local therapy consisting of compresses and sitz baths and the application of mild ointments designed to alleviate the inflammation. Even extensive networks of fistulas and abscesses can be cured with these local measures combined with bed rest, if necessary. Antibiotics are helpful in bacterial superinfection. Surgical measures such as the incision of a painful abscess should only be undertaken as a last resort during the florid stage of Crohn's disease. The excision of fistulas or fissures as well as the correction of stenoses is only indicated during phase of remission [2, 24, 26, 27, 64, 66, 125, 145, 169, 243, 249, 267, 268, 269, 272].

The most important diseases to consider in the differential diagnosis are venereal diseases such as chancroid, syphilis, and herpes simplex. The signs and symptoms, diagnosis and therapy of these diseases are described in the chapter on sexually transmitted anorectal diseases (pp. 142ff.).

Changes similar to those found in Crohn's disease are also seen in leukemia [274] and in tuberculosis. In leukemia, there are extensive necrotic lesions of the perianal skin, especially after local surgical procedures. Patients with open pulmonary tuberculosis can develop specific proctocolitis or perianal manifestations with sharply demarcated, painful ulcers with undermined edges and livid surrounding skin (Figure 320). Mycobacterium tuberculosis is identified by culture or by histological examination.

Therapy: Antituberculous drugs [15, 22, 58, 130, 246].

Changes similar to those of Crohn's disease are seen in Behçet's syndrome (Figures 321 and 322). Perianal ulcers, recurrent colitis resembling granulomatous Crohn's disease, and bouts of iridocyclitis are typical of this syndrome. It is accompanied less frequently by polyarthritis, thrombophlebitis, or erythema nodosum [51, 109].

Corticosteroids are recommended for therapy, followed by sulfasalazine, 5-aminosalicylic acid, and colchicine [169, 268].

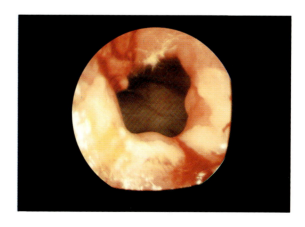

FIGURE 304
Stenosis of the anal canal due to fibrinous infiltration in a patient with regional colitis.

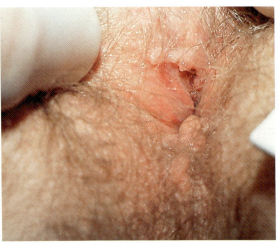

FIGURE 305
Ulcer in a patient with regional ileitis. To the left of the posterior midline there is a 5 by 10 mm ulcer with thick, edematous, irregular edges. It is not tender to touch.

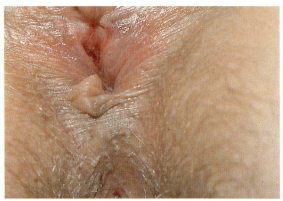

FIGURE 306
Anal ulcer under a sentinel pile in a patient with regional ileitis.

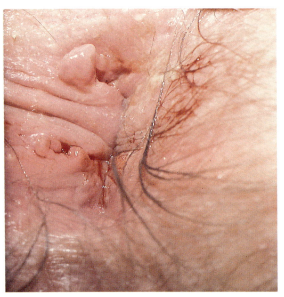

FIGURE 307
Ulcers in a patient with regional ileitis.

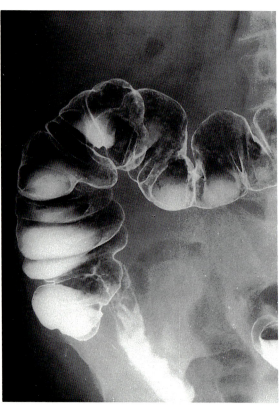

FIGURE 308
The same patient as in Figure 307: Typical radiological signs of terminal ileitis, such as stiffness of the terminal ileum and cobblestone pattern.

FIGURE 309–310

A fistula and an ulcer in a patient with regional ileitis .

There is an ulcer in the posterior midline. Foul-smelling pus is discharged when the buttocks are spread. The opening of a fistula is found 10 cm from the anus from which a small amount of yellowish pus is expelled during straining. Digital examination reveals a normal sphincter muscle tone, and on proctoscopy normal rectal mucosa is seen with its visible vascular network. Above the recto-sigmoid boundary the mucosa is thickened with ulceration and pus (see Figure 310). Epithelioid granulomas were found in the biopsy taken from the sigmoid colon confirming the diagnosis of regional enteritis (Institute of Pathology, Canton Hospital in St. Gallen).

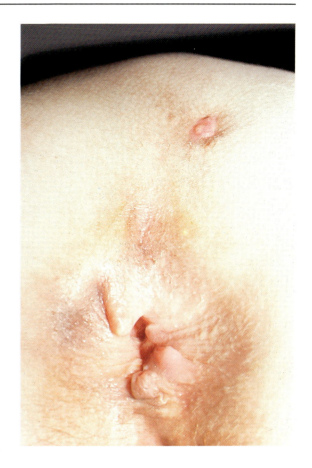

FIGURE 310

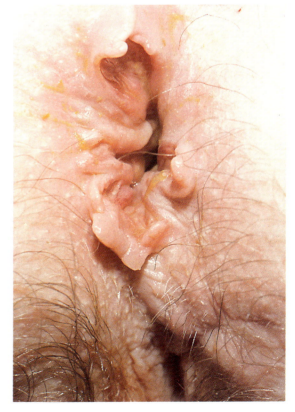

FIGURE 311
Ulcers in Crohn's disease.

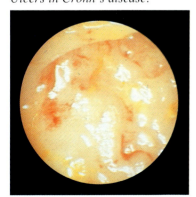

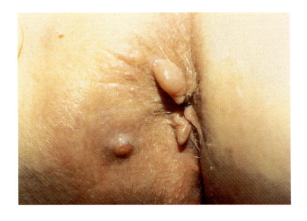

FIGURE 312
Edematous, suppurating skin tags in a patient with Crohn's disease of the ascending colon.

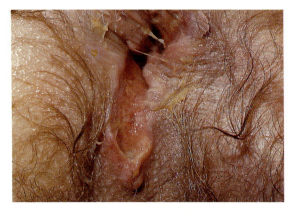

FIGURE 313
Extensive ulceration in the anterior and posterior midline in a patient with Crohn's disease of the descending colon.

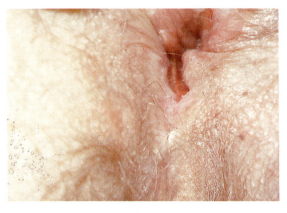

FIGURE 314
The same patient as in Figure 313 after 6 weeks of therapy with oral sulfasalazine. The ulcers are in the process of cicatrization.

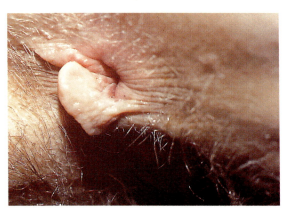

FIGURE 315
Edematous skin tags in a patient with regional enteritis of the descending colon.

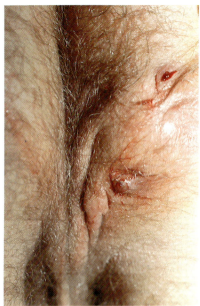

FIGURE 316
Perianal abscess and fistulas in a patient with regional enteritis. The perianal skin is reddened with scarring, and two fistula orifices are seen on the right.

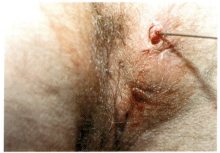

FIGURE 317
Two fistula tracts leading in different directions can be identified with a blunt probe.

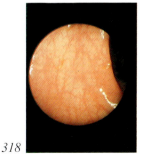
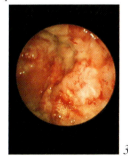

318   *319*

FIGURES 318 & 319
The diagnosis is confirmed by endoscopy. The rectal mucosa is pale pink and smooth with a well-defined submucosal vascular network (Figure 318), whereas the mucosa in the sigmoid colon is thickened with diffuse bleeding, purulent deposits and polyp-like mucosal changes (Figure319).

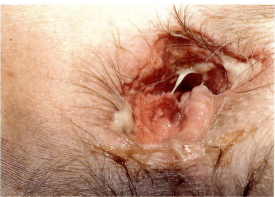

FIGURE 320
Skin ulceration in a patient with tuberculosis. Extensive and deep ulcerations in a patient with pulmonary and cecal tuberculosis.

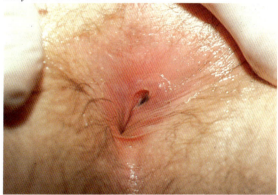

FIGURE 321
An ulcer in a patient with Behçet's syndrome.

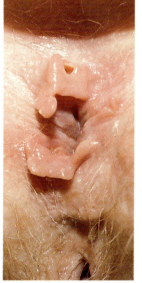
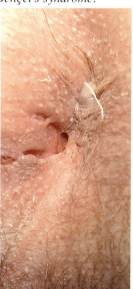

FIGURE 322
Right: Hidrosadenitis suppurativa (Verneuil): Anal ulcers and fistular orifices.
Left: Ulcers and skin tags with fistular orifices at the dorsal midline in a patient with lymphatic leukemia.

Specific Diseases with Defined Etiology

Radiation proctitis: Diarrhea and bleeding from hemorrhagic proctitis can occur weeks or even years after X-ray or radium therapy. The inflammatory lesions of the mucosa are located in the area of the former radiation field. In some cases, the blood loss can be severe enough to cause anemia and necessitate blood transfusions. Local therapy with suppositories or enemas containing corticosteroids or mesalazine can be beneficial [55, 76, 88, 107, 178, 179].

Infective proctitis: Acute diarrhea with bloody stools, tenesmus, and fever should alert one to the possibility of an infection with salmonella, shigella, campylobacter jejuni, or chlamydia [17, 75, 249, 261, 266, 270]. The proctological findings in these diseases are frequently indistinguishable from those of ulcerative colitis. In bacterial colitis the rectum is often spared so that proctoscopy alone is not enough to diagnose the cause of hemorrhagic colitis and will have to be supplemented with coloscopy. The diagnosis is confirmed by bacteriological and serological examination. A chronic course of the disease may indicate one of the rare cases of tuberculosis or actinomycosis.

Anorectal gonorrhea can cause the same lesions as a moderately active ulcerative colitis of the rectum. Since this disease usually occurs in homosexual men and less often in women, an accurate history can put one on the right diagnostic track. The diagnosis is made by identifying gonococci in the Gram-stained rectal swab or by culture. The therapy is described in the chapter on sexually transmitted diseases (pp. 142ff.).

In *anorectal syphilis*, the primary lesion is usually an ulcer located at the anorectal junction. In isolated cases, the primary lesion can be situated above the pectinate line causing a severe inflammatory infiltration of the submucosa resembling an ulcerated tumor. Nodular, indurated lesions of the rectal mucosa are also seen in secondary syphilis. The diagnosis is confirmed by serological examinations. The therapy is described in the chapter on sexually transmitted diseases (pp. 142ff.).

Proctitis from infection with chlamydia, often seen subsequent to anorectal gonorrhea, frequently causes narrowing of the rectum. The diagnosis is made by serological identification of chlamydia trachomatis.

Therapy: Tetracyclines should by given in a low dosage for an extended length of time to prevent recurrence. The recommended daily dosage for 10 to 15 days is tetracycline 2 g; doxycycline 200 mg; erythromycin 2 g [212].

Mycoplasms can act as pathogens in the same manner as chlamydia; they respond to the same therapy [223].

Herpes proctitis presenting as a purulent-hemorrhagic proctitis is commonly observed in homosexual males. Typical of this disease are severe pains in the rectum aggravated by defecation, tenesmus, and swollen inguinal lymph nodes. The identification of virus in cell culture confirms the diagnosis.

Therapy: Acyclovir is effective if initiated promptly [49, 249].

Proctitis can occur in AIDS (acquired immune deficiency syndrome). It can present as a simple erythema but aphthous lesions as well as purulent ulcerating forms are also observed. The lesions can extend into the sigmoid colon or can be confined to the cecum or sigmoid colon. The histological changes are intravascular thromboses and infiltration with cells showing cytomegalic inclusion bodies. Kaposi sarcomas are located not only on the skin, but also anywhere in the gastrointestinal tract as well as in the lungs.

AIDS is diagnosed by the demonstration of antibodies against the AIDS-virus (HIV). The test is not positive until 3 to 12 weeks after infection [13, 118, 216, 273].

Treatment: In some cases of cutaneous Kaposi sarcoma, interferon alpha-2a seems to be effective.

Actinomycosis: Actinomyces israelii can cause chronic anorectal inflammation with marked induration as well as abscesses and fistulas. The diagnosis is confirmed by the histological demonstration of grains ("sulphur granules") in biopsy material, or by bacteriological examination of pus. The pathogen responds favorably to high doses of penicillin [206].

Tuberculous proctocolitis can occur in patients suffering from open pulmonary tuberculosis or primary tuberculosis of the colon. This can cause painful perianal lesions with sharply demarcated ulcers and undermined edges. The identification of mycobacterium tuberculosis in cultured biopsies of colonic mucosa or in direct histological specimens confirms the diagnosis. The treatment is with antituberculor drugs [15, 22, 58, 96, 130, 219, 246] (see Figure 320).

Pseudomembranous enterocolitis (antibiotic-induced enterocolitis): This disorder occurs after treatment with antibiotics, either immediately or after a silent interval. Bloody diarrhea is seen together with fever and a rapid deterioration of the patient's general condition. Endoscopy should be performed as soon as possible after the onset of symptoms to confirm the diagnosis. One finds an inflamed, easily injured mucosa covered with white plaques and pseudomembranes. The white cell count is elevated both in blood and in stool, where they can be seen after staining with methylene blue. The symptoms usually disappear a few days after the antibiotics are discontinued. Treatment with loperamide, vancomycin, or corticosteroids is sometimes necessary [65, 102, 211, 236].

Parasites: Proctitis from parasites is observed in patients from tropic and subtropic countries. Acute schistosomiasis can resemble bacterial dysentery with bloody-mucoid diarrhea, tenesmus, and fever. The calcified ova can sometimes be felt as grains of sand in the mucosa during the rectal examination. The diagnosis is confirmed by the demonstration of ova in a biopsy of the rectal mucosa. The ova can also be found in the stool. The inflammatory lesions of the rectal mucosa disappear after treatment with niridazole (adults take 25 mg/kg bodyweight daily) [95, 249].

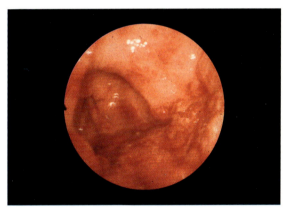

FIGURE 322a
Kaposi sarcoma. (This picture was kindly provided by Dr. Münch, Dept. of Internal Medicine, University Hospital, Zurich.)

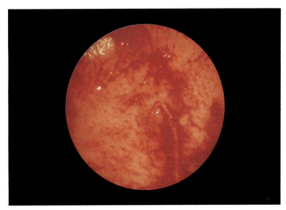

FIGURE 323
Hemorrhagic proctitis after X-ray therapy (radiation proctitis).

Amebiasis

Amebiasis is a disease of the tropics and sub-tropics which is being seen increasingly in temperate regions as a result of mass tourism.

Infection is acquired by ingesting in food or water the cysts of Entamoeba histolytica, which are the resistant form of the parasite, . In the human intestine, the cysts rupture releasing four trophozoites (amebas), which grow and multiply, usually existing as commensals without detrimental effects on their host. The trophozoites can encyst. Only certain strains of E. histolytica migrate into the tissues causing destruction and ulceration [85].

Symptoms: Diarrhea with blood and mucus occurs in acute cases. The mucus is transparent and the mixed blood gives it the appearance of raspberry jelly. Fever is absent in uncomplicated cases. In contrast to amebiasis, patients with bacillary dysentery have fever with more frequent and purulent stools. Intermittent diarrhea (with semifluid stool containing mucus) and constipation is the characteristic symptom of chronic amebiasis. Flatulence and bloating also occur.

Proctoscopy reveals normal mucosa with isolated small bleeding lesions typically located on mucosal folds, small ulcers with ragged, undermined edges and a greasy looking base which may become confluent. There is also increased production of mucus (Figures 325 and 326). In heavy infestations, amebiasis resembles ulcerative colitis when seen through the proctoscope, with a thick, velvety granular mucosa which bleeds on touch. Healing sometimes causes scar formation [138].

The diagnosis is confirmed by the demonstration of trophozoites in stool, mucus or tissues, or by serologic tests. Mucus is aspirated from the edge of an ulcer, transferred to a warm slide, mixed with a drop of isotonic saline, and immediately examined with an oil immersion objective. The trophozoites are mobile and extrude pseudopodia. The invasive form, i.e., the large form, contains phagocytized erythrocytes. The nucleus of the centrally located inclusion body is made visible by staining with Lugol's iodine. This rapidly causes a loss of mobility of the trophozoites. Stool samples are fixed in MIF (methiolate, iodine, formalin) or SAF (sodium acetate, acetic acid, formalin) prior to sending them to a special laboratory for examination. The diagnosis of invasive amebiasis can also be made by demonstrating antibodies by means of immunofluorescence, or hemagglutination or latex agglutination tests. These tests are positive in 60–80% of all patients with intestinal amebiasis and in 100% of patients with hepatic disease, while they usually give negative results in asymptomatic carriers.

Therapy: Cyst passers or patients with asymptomatic intestinal colonization should be treated with diloxanide furoate 500 mg orally 3 times daily for 10 days to avoid the risk of exacerbation or spread to extraintestinal organs. In uncomplicated amebiasis, metronidazole 500 mg 4 times daily is given for 3 to 5 days followed by diloxanide furoate. In severe cases of amebic dysentery, the combined therapy with metronidazole, tetracycline and perhaps dehydroemetine [245] is recommended.

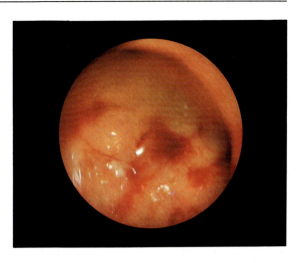

FIGURE 324
Spotty mucosal bleeding in a patient with amoebic dysentery. (This picture was kindly provided by Prof. Dr. med. W. Mohr, former head of the Clinical Department of the Bernhard-Nocht Institute in Hamburg.)

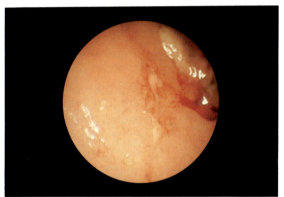

FIGURE 325
Amoebic dysentery with small ulcerations.

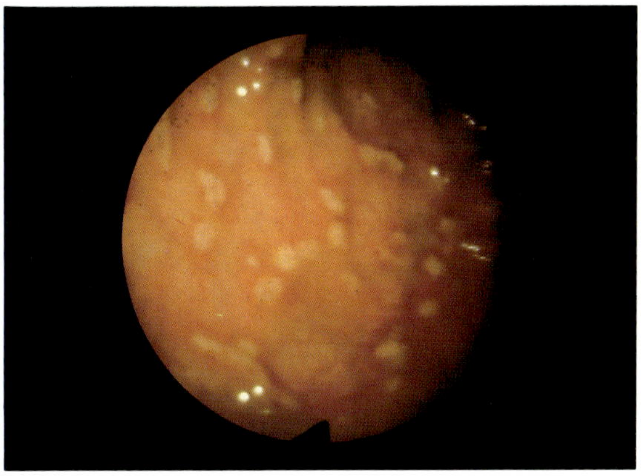

FIGURE 326
Amoebic dysentery with multiple ulcers. (Figures 325 and 326 were kindly provided by Prof. Dr. med. P. Kiefhaber, Head of the Department of Internal Medicine at the Municipal Hospital in Traunstein.)

Tumors of the Rectum

The incidence of both benign and malignant colon neoplasms decreases proximally from the rectum to the cecum.

Benign Tumors

The great majority of rectal tumors arise as polyps from the epithelium (hyperplastic polyps, juvenile polyps, adenomas). Mesenchymal tumors are rare (lipomas, hemangiomas, myomas). Further neoplastic lesions are the lymphoid polyps and others due to inflammation, as well as the hamartomatous polyps seen in Peutz-Jeghers syndrome and the polyps of the Cronkhite-Canada syndrome [74].

The most common benign tumors are epithelial neoplasms such as pedunculated, villous, or tubulovillous adenomas. These tumors are facultative precancerous lesions (WHO 1972). The risk of malignant transformation depends on the size and the histological differentiation of the adenoma. Adenomas larger than 2 cm with a villous histology are associated with a high risk.

Symptoms: Usually very few; occasionally slight to moderate bleeding. Large villous adenomas ("shaggy tumors") can cause severe loss of fluid and electrolytes.

Diagnosis: Macroscopic examination during endoscopy permits only an educated guess at the nature of the tumor. Histological examination of the entire tumor is the only sure way of confirming the diagnosis.

Therapy: All tumors discovered during endoscopy are removed and examined histologically. If a pedunculated polyp has severely dysplastic cells in the head, though without invasion of the stalk, then it is sufficient just to remove the polyp. If a carcinoma with a low or moderate degree of malignancy is located in the adenoma, then routine follow-up is sufficient as long as the resection boundary is free of malignant tissue. Segmental colon section is performed whenever there are tumor cells in the resection line, or the tumor is highly malignant, or when the tumor has penetrated a vessel.

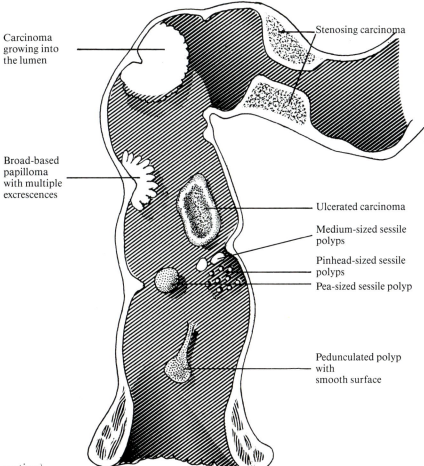

Carcinoma
growing into
the lumen

Stenosing carcinoma

Broad-based
papilloma
with multiple
excrescences

Ulcerated carcinoma

Medium-sized sessile
polyps

Pinhead-sized sessile
polyps

Pea-sized sessile polyp

Pedunculated polyp
with
smooth surface

FIGURE 327
Tumors of the rectum (sagittal section).

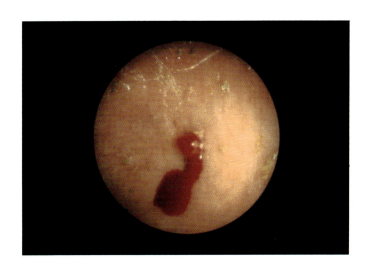

FIGURE 328
Small bleeding hyperplastic polyp.

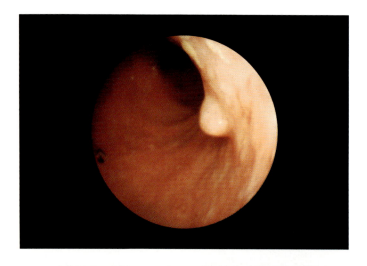

FIGURE 329
Sessile, hyperplastic polyp.

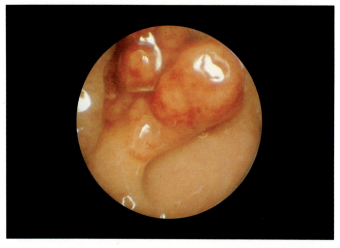

FIGURE 330
Pedunculated polyp in the rectum.

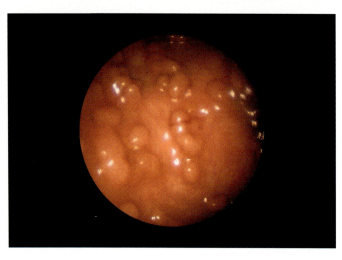

FIGURE 331
Polyposis of the rectum.

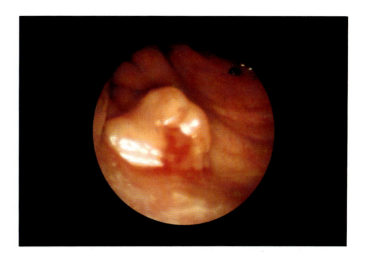

FIGURE 332
Bleeding sessile adenoma.

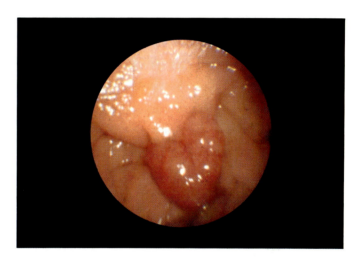

FIGURE 333
Sessile villous adenoma.

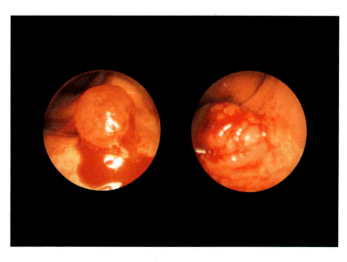

FIGURE 334
Left: bleeding hyperplastic rectal polyp;
right: bleeding tubulovillous adenoma.

128

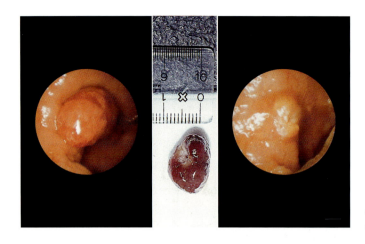

FIGURE 335
Benign tumor after cautery resection.

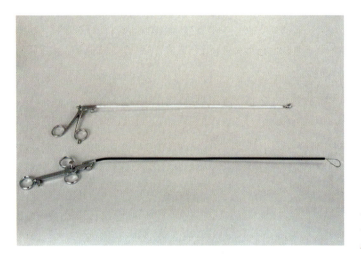

FIGURE 336
Biopsy forceps, cautery snare for removing pedunculated tumors.

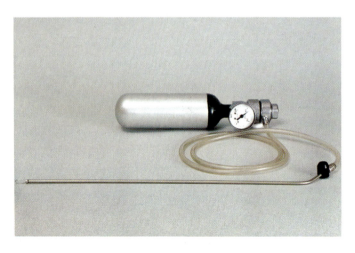

FIGURE 337
Tank of nitrogen connected to a metal tube. This is used to displace the methane from the colon and the proctoscope before cautery to prevent explosions.

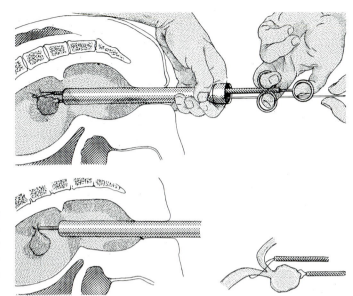

FIGURE 338
Removing benign tumors with the cautery snare. The snare is looped around the tumor, which is removed at its base under gentle traction. If the traction on the tumor is too strong there is the risk of perforating the wall (lower right).

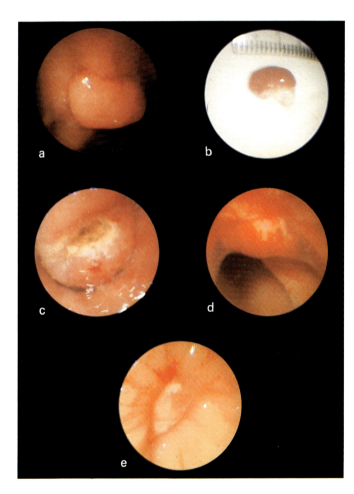

FIGURE 339
Polyp before and after removal with the cautery snare:
a) Polyp in situ
b) Polyp after removal with the cautery snare
c) Site of coagulation immediately after electroresection
d) Scarring 1 month later
e) Scarring 1 year later.

Polyposis Syndromes

Polyposis syndromes can arise in the entire gastrointestinal tract, and thus also in the rectum. They are rare, but they can pose diagnostic and therapeutic difficulties. The syndromes can be classified into non-neoplastic and neoplastic categories. Neoplastic polyposis (adenomatosis) are regarded as obligate precancerous lesions (WHO 1972) [29, 74, 235, 259].

- A. *Non-neoplastic polyposis*
  Juvenile polyposis
  Peutz-Jeghers syndrome
  Cowden's syndrome
  Cronkhite-Canada syndrome
  Benign lymphoid polyposis

- B. *Neoplastic polyposis*
  Familial polyposis
  Gardner' syndrome
  Turcot's syndrome

Nonneoplastic Polyposis

Juvenile polyposis appears between the ages of 5 and 9. Pedunculated polyps with a diameter of 3 to 20 mm with a smooth surface are observed. The polyps disappear during puberty. A low risk of malignant transformation is presumed [20, 152, 209, 210, 249].

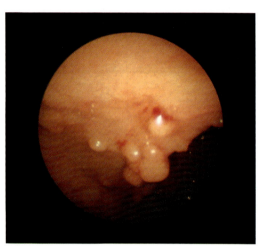

FIGURE 340
Smooth tumors projecting into the lumen of the gut in a patient with juvenile polyposis. There are isolated spots of bleeding at the bases.

Peutz-Jeghers Syndrome

Small deposits of melanin on the nose, the lips, and the buccal mucosa are typical for the Peutz-Jeghers syndrome. The spots are found less often on the extensor sides of the elbows and the interphalangal joints. A further feature is the occurrence of intestinal polyps located anywhere from the stomach to the rectum, but most commonly found in the small intestine. This predilection for the highly mobile small intestine can be the cause of intussusception with crampy abdominal pains. Occult bleeding from the polyps can cause secondary anemia.

The syndrome occurs most frequently in patients under the age of 30. The polyps, which are considered to be hamartomas, have a stroma rich in muscle fibers that arises from the tunica muscularis propria and mucosae and includes neural elements. Malignant transformation has not been proven, and extensive prophylactic colon resections are not necessary [104].

Cowdon's Syndrome (Multiple Hamartomas)

This is a rare, autosomal-dominant, hereditary disease that appears in the second decade. The polyps are usually nonneoplastic and exhibit great variability with regards to number, size and localization.

Cronkhite-Canada Syndrome

Diarrhea and weight loss combined with hypoproteinemia and disturbed fluid and electrolyte balance are prominent features of the Cronkhite-Canada syndrome. Nonmalignant polyps are found from the gastric cardia to the rectum [39, 121].

Benign Lymphoid Polyposis

Hyperplasia of multiple solitary lymph nodes in the mucosa and submucosa can cause polyposis with multiple small, round polyps. Histology reveals that the enlarged solitary lymph follicles often contain the germinal centers that differentiate them from malignant follicular lymphomas of the intestine, which are less common.

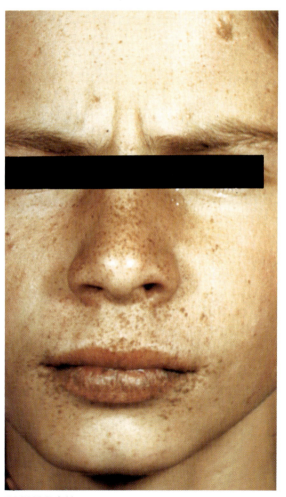

FIGURE 341
Distinctive facial pigmentation in a patient with Peutz-Jeghers syndrome.

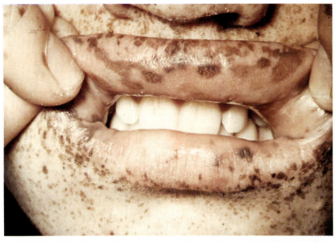

FIGURE 342
Pigmentation of the oral mucosa in a patient with Peutz-Jeghers syndrome.

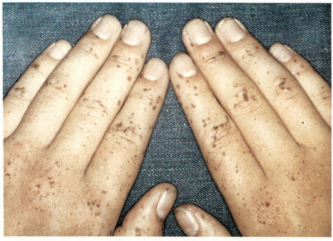

FIGURE 343
The pigmented spots are grouped over the finger joints.

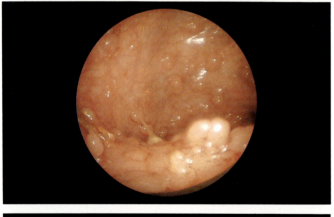

FIGURE 344
Rectal polyp in a patient with Peutz-Jeghers syndrome.

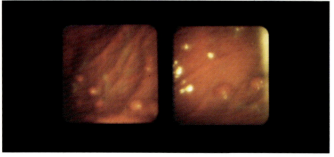

FIGURE 345
Polyp in the stomach of a patient with Peutz-Jeghers syndrome.

Neoplastic Polyposis

– Familial Adenomatous

This rare, dominantly transmitted disease is regarded as a precancerous condition. Diarrhea mixed with mucus is present and can lead to dehydration and electrolyte disturbances. The tumors usually appear during puberty. The rectum and colon may contain relatively few polyps, but they also can be totally overgrown with them. They may be interspersed with solitary pedunculated adenomas. The tendency toward malignant transformation is high—virtually every patient with familial polyposis develops cancer of the colon by the age of 40, so that early total colectomy and proctectomy is the therapy of choice. Nine percent of the patients develop desmoid tumors that show local infiltrative growth and can cause severe abdominal complications.

– Gardner's Syndrome

This is a type of polyposis with a strong tendency toward malignant transformation associated with mesenchymal tumors of other organs. Besides the disseminated intestinal polyps, other mesenchymal tumors are also found, such as fibromas, cutaneous lipomas, and osteomas of the maxilla, the skull, and long bones.

– Turcot's Syndrome

This is a combination of neoplasms of the central nervous system and familial polyposis. It is extremely rare and is transmitted as an autosomal recessive disorder.

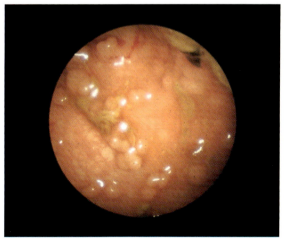

FIGURE 346
Familial polyposis. (Figures 344–346 were kindly provided by Prof. Dr. med. C. F. Klistermann of the Dermatological Clinic of the University of Göttingen.)

Intestinal Pneumatosis (Pneumatosis cystoides intestinalis)

In this disorder, one finds groups of 1 to 20 mm large, gas-containing cysts in the wall of the small intestine and colon. The lesions are usually submucosal in young patients and subserosal in older patients. Serial histological sections reveal communicating systems filled with gas with the same composition as the atmosphere.

This is a benign condition that usually disappears by itself in a matter of days or weeks but which can recur.

Diagnosis: is based on the radiological demonstration of translucent spots arranged like pearls on a string. Round mucosal bumps that look like transparent sessile polyps are seen during proctoscopy. These collapse if a biopsy is attempted (which it shouldn't be).

Symptoms: unspecific abdominal pains, pronounced constipation, rarely diarrhea, and passage of blood or mucus. Occasionally, a cyst can rupture and cause an acute pneumoperitoneum.

Treatment: is necessary only in cases of bloody or mucoid diarrhea. In these instances, neomycin or bismuth is recommended. Resection of the affected section of intestine is necessary only for complications such as obstruction or infection. Severe symptoms can be treated with oxygen in an oxygen tent, mask, or hyperbaric oxygen therapy [62].

Etiology: A mechanistic theory holds that intestinal gas is pressed through a valve-like lesion in the intestinal wall [13]. Another theory, which is supported by animal experiments, claims that in pulmonary diseases respiratory air escapes from ruptured alveoles into the mediastinum and passes retroperitoneally from there along the course of vessels into the intestinal wall [14, 32, 35, 52, 108].

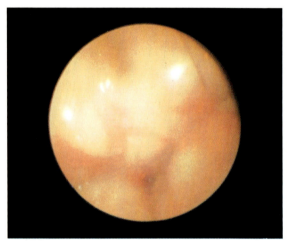

FIGURE 347
10mm large cysts in intestinal pneumatosis (pneumatosis cystoides intestinalis).

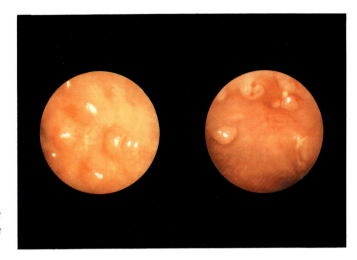

FIGURE 348
Left: mucosal bulges in cystic pneumatosis
intestinalis; right: bleeding rectal polyps in
comparison.

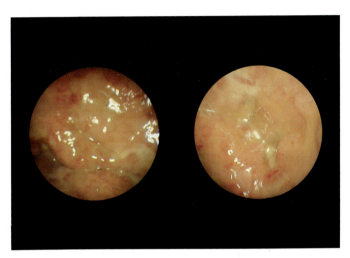

FIGURE 349
Lobulated bulge of rectal mucosa in cystic
pneumatosis intestinalis.

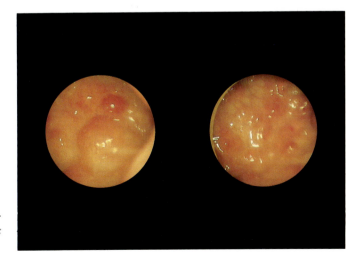

FIGURE 350
Lobulated bulge of edematous rectal mu-
cosa which is coated with blood and pus
(cystic pneumatosis intestinalis)

Malignant Tumors

These are usually adenocarcinomas and, less frequently, signet-ring cell carcinomas. Mesenchymal neoplasms such as myosarcomas or lymphomas are extremely rare.

Epithelial neoplasms (adenomas), ulcerative colitis of the entire colon lasting for more than ten years, and Crohn's disease of the colon are facultative precancerous lesions. Familial polyposis is an obligatory precancerous condition.

Symptoms: Bleeding, either massive or trace, anemia due to blood loss, sensation of fullness in the rectum, spurious urge to defecate, altered bowel habit, especially diarrhea or tenesmus [159, 198].

Therapy: Resection or proctectomy. Small carcinomas can be treated by local excision [44, 78, 84, 133, 173, 174] or by direct-contact irradiation [16, 148, 184, 185, 188, 197, 199, 201, 202, 283] if they are mobile on palpation and not attached to lower structures, and if they have been shown to be localized to the mucosa by sonography and/or computerized tomography. Regular follow-up examination by endoscopy with biopsy, computerized tomography, and determinations of carcinoembryonal antigen (CEA) are necessary. Inoperable carcinomas can be partially removed by electro- or laser coagulation, or by cryotherapy [99, 146]. In individual cases, radiation therapy can render large tumors operable. Chemotherapy can have a beneficial effect on the subjective complaints.

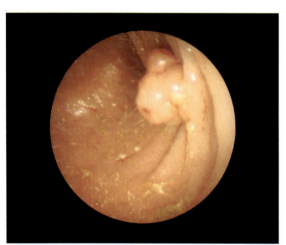

FIGURE 351
Small, partially pedunculated adenocarcinoma.

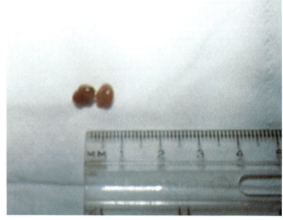

FIGURE 352
The tumor split in two after removal with the electric snare.

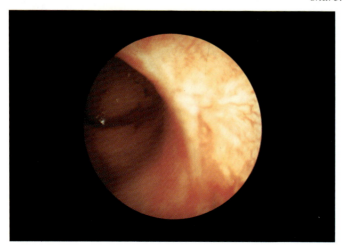

FIGURE 353
The same patient as in Figure 351 after ablation with 10,000 r radiation.

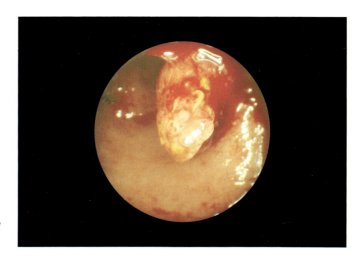

FIGURE 354
Exophytic adenocarcinoma in the rectal ampulla.

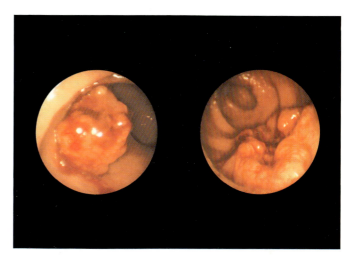

FIGURE 355
Left: exophytic adenocarcinoma; right: excavated adenocarcinoma at the rectosigmoid junction.

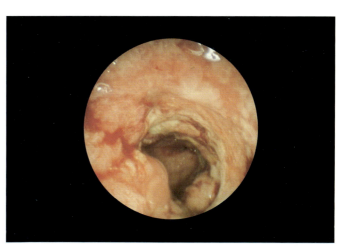

FIGURE 356
Adenocarcinoma causing obstruction of the rectum.

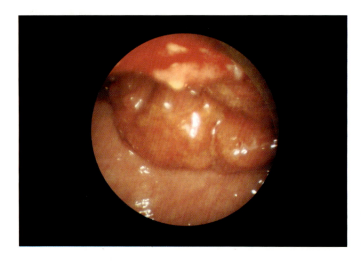

FIGURE 357
Sessile, exophytic adenocarcinoma of the rectum.

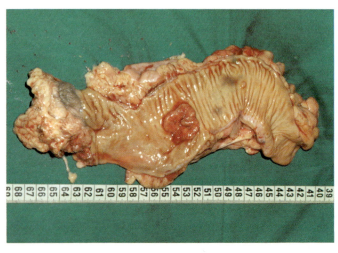

FIGURE 358
Pathologic specimen from the patient in Figure 357. A more restorative resection is usual.

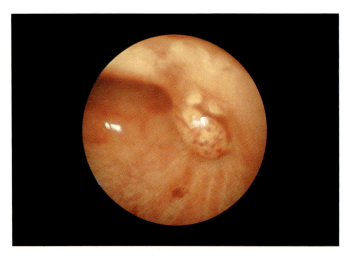

FIGURE 359
Foreign body granuloma at the site of the anastomosis 4 months after resection of an adenocarcinoma (granulomatous nature confirmed by histology).

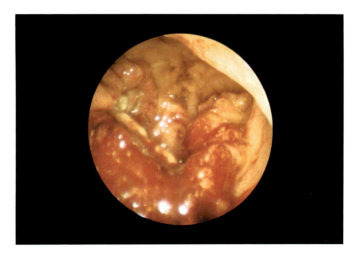

FIGURE 360
Extensive, ulcerated adenocarcinoma of the
rectum.

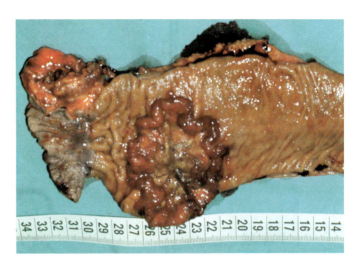

FIGURE 361
Pathologic specimen of the patient in Fig-
ure 360. Too low for restorative resection.

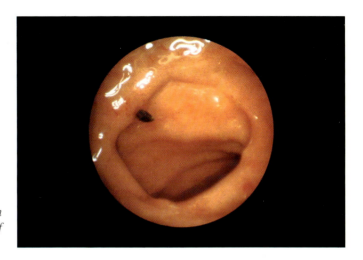

FIGURE 362
Black suture at site of anastomosis 16 cm
above the anus, 2 months after removal of
the rectal carcinoma.

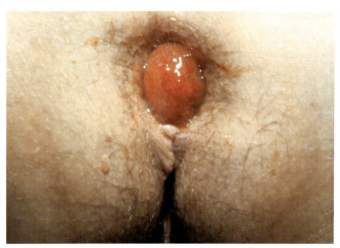

FIGURE 363
Pedunculated rectal carcinoma prolapsing through the anus.

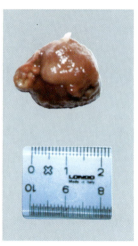

FIGURE 364
The tumor after electro-surgical removal.

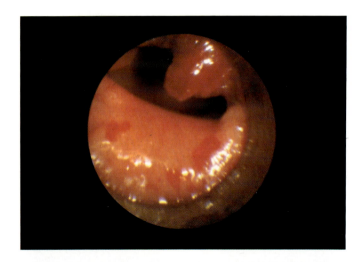

FIGURE 365
Small, mobile rectal carcinoma 8 cm above the anus.

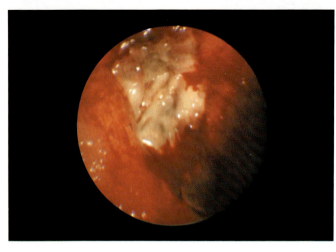

FIGURE 366
Necrotic area of mucosa 2 months after start of endorectal contact irradiation of the tumor with a total radiation dose of 8000 r.

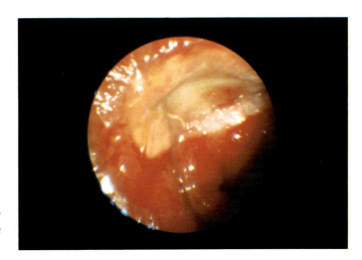

FIGURE 367
The same patient 6 months after beginning
of radiation therapy. Whitish scars are seen
on the mucosa.

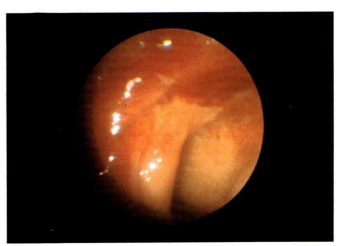

FIGURE 368
Scarred area with vascularization of the
surrounding tissue 1 year later [283].

Sexually Transmitted Anorectal Diseases

Genital warts (condylomata acuminata) caused by papilloma viruses, are the most common sexually transmitted disease. This is followed in frequency by syphilis, gonorrhea, genital herpes, chancroid, as well as infections with chlamydia and mycoplasmas. The perianal lesions associated with genital warts, syphilis, herpes and chancroid are so typical that they are usually recognized without difficulty. Sexually transmitted rectal diseases, on the other hand, are easily overlooked, since they present a clinical picture resembling ulcerative colitis. Swollen lymph nodes in the groin may indicate syphilis or chancroid [13, 31, 59, 60, 67, 113, 114, 183, 196, 208, 224, 225, 249, 257].

Syphilis

The primary lesion of syphilis, which appears about three weeks after infection, can be located near the anus or less frequently in the lower rectum. This should be kept in mind during the diagnostic work-up of atypical ulcers. Although this primary chancre is usually painless, it occasionally presents as an extremely painful anal fissure. Anal and rectal lesions are usually accompanied by foul-smelling secretions. The associated enlarged lymph nodes are located in the abdomen and in both groins.

The diagnosis of syphilis is confirmed by the detection of spirochetes (treponema pallidum) in the exudate from the primary lesion or in needle-biopsy specimens from swollen lymph nodes. Experience is needed in taking the specimens, which are examined by darkfield microscopy. The spirochetes are seen as fine, filiform, white coils, and recognized by their corkscrew rotation and angulation.

The specific serological tests, FTA (fluorescent treponemal antibody) and TPHA (treponema pallidum hemagglutination) are used to detect antitreponemal antibodies in the patient's blood. These tests usually become positive within 3 weeks after infection. When treatment is initiated in the primary or early secondary stage, the positive reaction can disappear. In most cases, however, the tests remain positive for the life of the patient in spite of effective therapy [135]. The diagnosis of active syphilis in a patient with long-standing positive seroreaction is made by demonstrating specific antitreponemal IgM antibodies. These disappear after the disease has healed.

Eight weeks after infection, untreated syphilis enters the secondary stage. The local infection becomes a generalized one, and macular and/or papular cutaneous eruptions (syphilids) appear. Papules developing in moist areas of skin, such as the perianal region, can become hypertrophic and flattened usually with exudation. These are termed condylomata lata and contain large numbers of spirochetes. Positive serological tests signify generalized infection.

Late or tertiary syphilis develops three to five years after infection and is characterized by cutaneous lesions (tuberoserpiginous syphilid) or subcutaneous knobs with a rubbery consistency (gummas), both of which tend to ulcerate. Kidney-shaped, punched-out ulcers are typical. The manifestations of tertiary syphilis may also appear in the perianal or gluteal region.

Treatment, formerly with penicillin (plus probenecid) requires ceftriaxone, spectinomycin, doxycycline, erythromycine or quilonines.

Gonorrhea

In males, rectal gonorrhea is almost exclusively caused by anal intercourse and is only rarely the sequel of a ruptured gonorrheal abscess of the prostate. In females, on the other hand, it is caused fairly frequently by infectious vaginal discharge.

The *symptoms*, such as itching, inflammation of the anus, and pain on defecation, are usually mild, but in severe cases the the disease can present with acute ulcerating proctitis and rectitis complicated by the formation of abscesses and fistulas. On endoscopy, one finds a more or less erythematous and edematous mucosa with patches of purulent secretions. Pus can frequently be expressed from the anal crypts.

The *diagnosis* is confirmed by identification of gonococci in stained smears and in culture. Specimens are gathered on anoscopy with a wire loop or cotton swabs. The intestinal mucosal exudate is spread on two slides and heat-fixated over a flame. One slide is stained for 15 seconds with a 1% aqueous solution of methylene blue, and the other with Gram's method. The coffee-bean shaped, gram-negative diplococci are found intra- and extracellularly in characteristic clumps.

Specimens for culture are also gathered with a loop or swab through the anoscope. If laboratory facilities are not immediately available, the specimens can be mailed in transport medium supplied by external laboratories.

Gonococcal antigens can also be demonstrated in specimens by enzyme immunoassay (EIA).

Treatment: Owing to frequent penicillase-producing gonococci the traditional combination of aqueous penicillin, amoxycillin or ampicillin with probenecid has been abandoned in favor of cephalosporins such as ceftriaxone, spectinomycin, doxycycline, erythromycine or the newer quinolines. The last three are also effective against Chlamydia trachomatis.

Herpes

Symptoms: The incubation period is four to five days. Intense pain and tenesmus occurs, which is aggravated by defecation. The inguinal lymph nodes are frequently enlarged. This is followed by disturbed micturition, sacral parasthesias and lumbar pain. Vesicles and ulcers are located around the anus, while irregular, highly inflamed, ulcerated patches covered with sanguineous purulent discharge are seen in the rectum.

The *diagnosis* is made by identifying the herpes simplex virus in serum from vesicles, swabs from mucosal ulcers or in biopsy material by its cytopathic effects in tissue culture. Histology reveals degenerative lesions of the mucosa. Herpes antigens can also be demonstrated directly by immunofluorescence.

Early *treatment* with Acyclovir is effective, and above all can prevent complications [90, 225, 249, 254, 257].

Chancroid (Soft Chancre)

This very rare disease is characterized by 1 to 2 cm large, soft, painful ulcers with ragged undermined edges which arise at the site of infection one to three days after exposition. Anal lesions are caused by anal intercourse. A frequent complication is a painful, regional lymphadenitis and perilymphadenitis rapidly leading to formation of a fluctuating abscess (bubo), which then penetrates the skin. If left untreated, lymph node abscesses and fistulas can develop.

The *diagnosis* is based on the demonstration of haemophilus ducreyi in material taken from the undermined edge on an ulcer. The Ito-Reenstierna test (positive reaction to the intracutaneous injection of specific haemophilus ducreyi antigen) is a further method.

The *treatment* of choice for chancroid is with tetracyclines, sulfonamides, or other antibiotics, such as streptomycin. To avoid masking concurrent syphilis, drugs should be used that are ineffective against treponema, such as sulfonamides [224, 249, 257].

Granuloma Inguinale (Granuloma Venereum)

This mildly contagious disease found predominantly in the tropics and subtropics is caused by the encapsulated bacteria Donovania granulomatis (calymmatobacterium granulomatis). It has been introduced into temperate climates as a result of mass tourism. Common sites of infection are the genital and inguinal regions, but it may also occur around the anus and in the rectum. The initial pustules and papules develop into luxurient, cauliflower-like growths that bleed easily. If left untreated, the disease persists for years. Scar formation can cause gross mutilation of the genital organs and the rectum. The diagnosis is confirmed by the identification of the causative organism in the foul-smelling secretions.

Treatment is with tetracyclines or other broad spectrum antibiotics and should begin as early as possible. Local corrective surgical measures should be considered in advanced disease [178, 225, 249, 257].

Lymphogranuloma Venereum (lymphogranuloma Inguinale, lymphopathia Venereum, Nicolas-Favre Disease)

This disease, also known as the fifth venereal disease, is found mostly in tropical and subtropical areas, and is caused by certain strains of chlamydia trachomatis. Since the usual means of transmission is by sexual intercourse, the primary lesions are seen in the genital area and only occasionally in the anus or on the tongue or fingers.

At the earliest a week after infection, an initial atypical ulcer appears the size of a grain of rice. Later the regional lymph nodes (usually the inguinal nodes) swell and coalesce to form large masses that adhere to the overlying erythematous skin, break down and perforate, frequently forming sinuses.

A particularly unpleasant complication involves a complex of anorectal symptoms that can be recognized by the perianal masses. Involvement of perirectal lymphatics causes infiltration and thickening of the rectal wall which obstructs the lumen to such an extent that only small-caliber "pencil" stools can pass. Rectal ulcers and perianal and perirectal fistulas can also develop. Urethral strictures as well as urethrovaginal and vaginorectal fistulas are not uncommon in females. Extensive destruction of pelvic lymphatics may result in genital elephantiasis.

The diagnosis is confirmed by the identification of chlamydia in the purulent discharge from a bubo, immunofluorescent staining with antichlamydial antibodies, the Frei intradermal test (positive reaction with erythema, pustules or necrosis within 48 hours after intracutaneous injection of Chlamydia antigen), or demonstration of IgG and IgA antibodies against chlamydia trachomatis in the patient's blood.

The disease is treated with tetracyclines or other broad-spectrum antibodies and should begin as early as possible. Local corrective surgical measures should be considered in advanced disease [136].

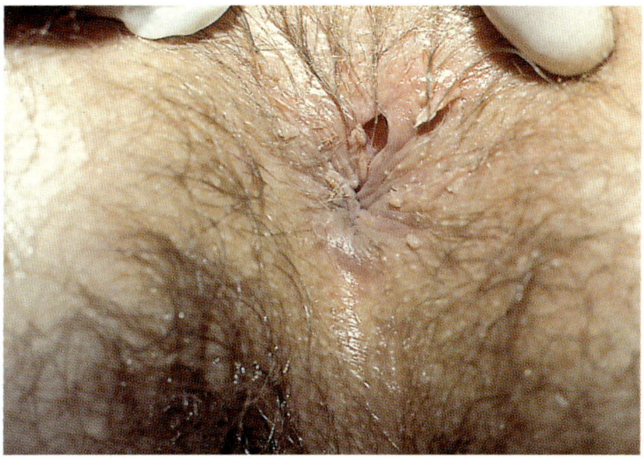

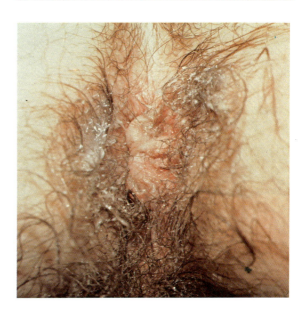

FIGURE 369
Condylomata acuminata and primary chancre in the
posterior midline.

FIGURE 370
Broad perianal tumorous lesions with sero-positive
condylomata lata (secondary syphilis).

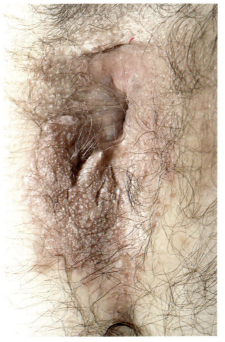

FIGURE 371
Condylomata lata. Flattened papules with a granu-
lar surface to the right of and posterior to the anus.
A positive serological test confirmed the diagnosis of
secondary syphilis (see also Figure 213).

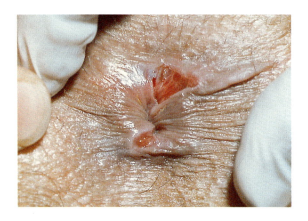

FIGURE 372
Syphilitic chancres in the anterior and posterior midline (primary syphilis).

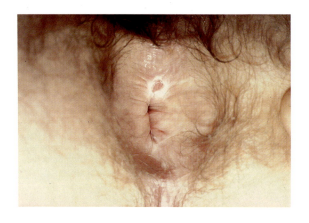

FIGURE 373
Chancre in the posterior midline (primary syphilis).

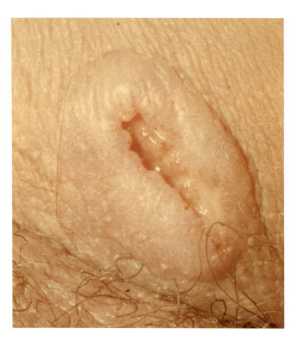

FIGURE 374
Inguinal gumma (tertiary syphilis). The illustration was kindly provided by Dr. I. Lentini from the Centro Proctologica in Barcelona.

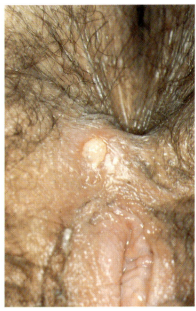

FIGURE 375
Chancroid. The illustration was kindly provided by
Prof. T. Rufli from the Dermatological Department
of the University Hospital in Basel.

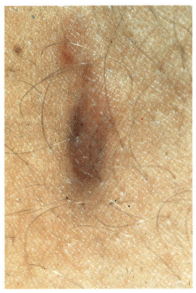

FIGURE 376
Kaposi sarcoma. The illustration was kindly pro-
vided by Dr. med. M. Flepp from the Department for
Infectious Diseases at the University Hospital for
Internal Medicine in Zurich.

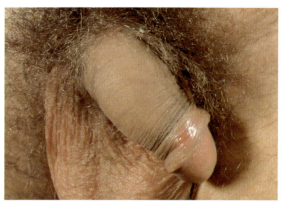

FIGURE 377
Lymphogranuloma venereum with an ulcer on the
glans penis. The illustration was kindly provided by
Prof. T. Rufli from the Dermatological Department
of the University Hospital in Basel.

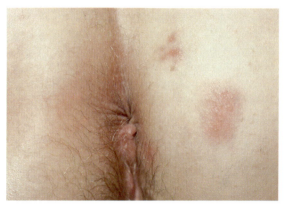

FIGURE 378
Herpes vesicles on the right buttock.

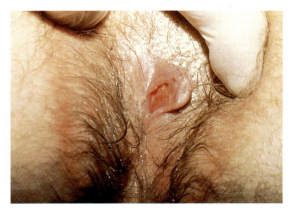

FIGURE 379
Genital herpes simplex infection with an ulcer to the
right of the posterior midline.

Sigmoidoscopy and Colonoscopy

It is frequently not possible to diagnose conditions of the sigmoid colon by double-contrast radiography alone because of the anatomic peculiarities such as the convoluted shape and the superimposition of segments. The examination with a flexible fiberoptic endoscope and biopsy can be of considerable help in such cases [33, 36, 63, 64, 112, 149, 171, 178, 231, 277].

The common indications for endoscopy are for diagnosis of bleeding of unknown origin, polyps, the differentiation of diverticulosis with inflammatory alterations of the bowel wall from infiltrative malignant processes, and therapeutic procedures such as electric snare removal of pedunculated polyps. Endoscopy is contraindicated in patients with fulminant colitis and acute diverticulitis.

amination. The rigid anoscope is better for inspecting the anal canal than the thin fiberscope.

A hinged anoscope with a glass-fiber light source for the preliminary anoscopy has been developed by TREIER (see Figure 380). After anoscopy, it is used as an introducer for the fiberoptic instrument. Once the latter is inserted, the anoscope is withdrawn from the anal canal, opened, and removed.

The main complication of colonooscopy is perforation of the bowel wall [100, 151, 281]. In a survey conducted in 27 gastroenterological centers by FRÜHMORGEN, an incidence of 0.14% was reported. Bleeding occurred in 0.008%, and the mortality was 0.02% [70].

Procedure

The fiberoptic colonoscope, which has a separate channel for biopsy and electrosurgical instruments, is introduced with the patient in the left lateral position. Under constant vision and occasionally with fluoroscopic control, it is guided through the rectum and sigmoid colon and advanced until it reaches the cecum. The lumen is kept open by inflation with air and the bowel is inspected both during insertion and removal of the instrument.

The bowel must by completely empty before the examination. Cathartics containing senna or cascara, administered the day before the examination, are suitable agents. The patients are also required to drink at least two liters of fluids and not to eat solid foods. If the bowel is not completely empty, a high enema can be given 1 hour before the examination.

Careful inspection of the anal region, digital examination of the anal canal, and anoscopy must be performed prior to the fiberoptic ex-

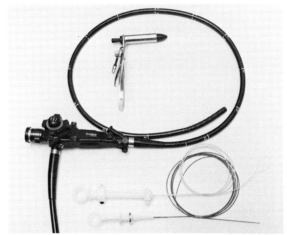

FIGURE 380
Flexible fiberoptic sigmoidocoloscope used for the Figures 381–387, 389 and 390 (Fujinon COL-M) with biopsy forceps and electric snare.
Hinged anoscope with a connector for the glass-fiber light cable (Manufactured by R. Treier, CH-6215 Beromünster, Switzerland).

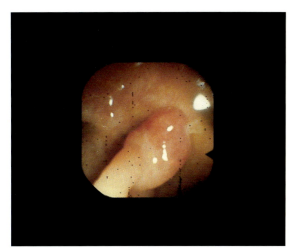

FIGURE 381
Hyperplastic, pedunculated mucosal polyp in the sigmoid colon.

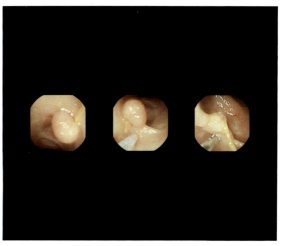

FIGURE 382
Papillary adenoma in the sigmoid colon seen before, during, and after electrosurgical removal.

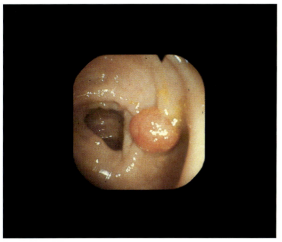

FIGURE 383
Papillovillous adenoma in the sigmoid colon.

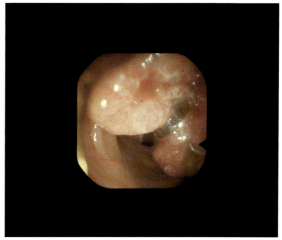

FIGURE 384
Adenocarcinoma in the sigmoid colon.

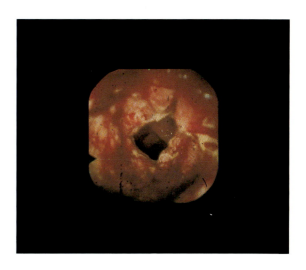

FIGURE 385
Adenocarcinoma in the sigmoid colon obstructing the lumen.

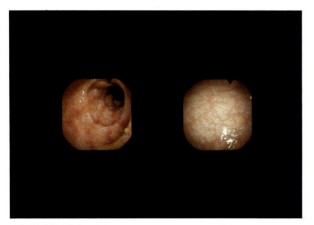

FIGURE 386
Left: Lesions of regional enteritis in the sigmoid colon with bleeding, edematous mucosa. Right: The rectal mucosa is unaffected; it is pink, smooth and with a normal vascular pattern.

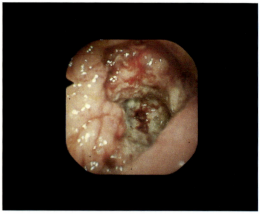

FIGURE 387
Extensive carcinoma tubulare et pailliferum of the cecum.

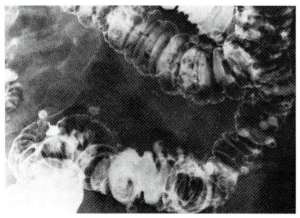

FIGURE 388
Radiograph of a 63-year-old patient with extensive diverticulosis of the sigmoid colon.

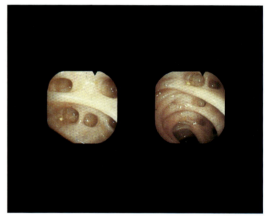

FIGURE 389
Endoscopic view of the colonic diverticula with normal mucosa and vascular pattern (the same patient as in Figure 388).

Diverticulosis of the Sigmoid Colon

Diverticulosis is characterized by mucosal herniations through the muscular wall of the colon at the entry sites of the colonic blood vessels and through gaps in the longitudinal musculature. The herniations occur most often when the intraluminal pressure is increased. They are most common in the sigmoid colon since here the intraluminal pressure can be two to five times higher than in the other portions of the colon.

Symptoms: Uncomplicated diverticulosis is usually asymptomatic. Half of the patients with diverticula never have complaints, but because of the possible complications they should be informed of their existence.

Complications: Retention of fecal matter in the diverticula can cause acute inflammation. The diverticulitis can spread to surrounding structures causing peridiverticulitis, which can simulate left-sided appendicitis. Perforation is not uncommon, and small abscesses can penetrate into the intestinal lumen. The diverticulum can be obliterated by fibrotic processes after a bout of inflammation. The inflammation can be recurrent or chronic.

The symptoms of the complications are sensation of pressure, pain, and cramps in the left lower quadrant, which are aggravated by defecation, external pressure or certain movements. An abscess can penetrate into a mesenterial vein causing portal bacteremia with chills and spiking fever. The peripheral blood culture is usually negative, since the bacteria are removed by the liver.

The clinical examination may reveal a tender cylindrical mass in the left lower abdomen. Endoscopy should not be performed in acute cases because of the danger of perforation.

Perforation into the free peritoneal cavity is rare, since it is usually walled off. Bladder pain may indicate perforation into the bladder. Bowel obstruction from edema is reversible, but may become permanent because of fibrosis in chronic disease. In this case, resection may be indicated, especially to exclude the possibility of an obstructive carcinoma. Carcinoma is not more common in patients with diverticulosis, but a tumor obstructing the lumen can predispose to diverticulosis and diverticulitis.

In 20–30% of the cases, bleeding is the sole clinical manifestation. It arises from erosions at the base of a diverticulum and can be very profuse. It can be localized by coloscopy, or by angiography if the blood loss is more than 0.5 to 1 ml per minute. Bleeding usually stops spontaneously, and surgical treatment is only rarely necessary.

Acute bouts are treated with bed rest, fasting, intravenous fluids, broad-spectrum antibiotics, analgesics and spasmolytics, such as atropin, and glucagon to reduce colonic motility. Drastic laxatives should not be given. After the acute phase has subsided, the bowel habits are regulated with a high bulk diet containing bran, whole-meal bread, vegetables, fruit, and with bulk laxatives and fecal softeners. Hot spices and fruit with tiny seeds should be avoided [1, 41, 63, 140, 177, 178, 179, 193].

Ischemic colitis

The main localization is in the descending colon, especially in the splenic flexure; only rarely is the rectum involved. Venous congestion leads to the development of polypoid, blue-black protuberances that then progress to present the typical picture of pseudomembranous colitis with grayish-white to gray-black membranes consisting of blood, mucus, fibrin, and pus. The lesions are usually patchy and are limited by the tunica muscularis. The disease may heal with a return to normal or may lead to stenosis. Gangrene of the bowel occurs if complete ischemia affects the entire circumference.

Attacks can be precipitated by a drop in blood pressure with reduced circulation in the region supplied by the inferior mesenteric artery as in myocardial infarction, congestive heart failure, or traumatic shock. The diameter of the occluded vessel, the duration of occlusion, collateral circulation and the bacterial content of the intestine are decisive factors for the extent of the lesion.

Common symptoms are crampy left abdominal pain, frequently with vomiting, bloody diarrhea without signs of shock, and guarding. Acute diverticulitis is a differential diagnostic possibility. The endoscopic findings resemble those of ulcerative colitis with whitish-gray-bluish necrosis and livid discoloration of surrounding tissue.

The symptoms recede within a few days. During the first days, radiography reveals segmental narrowing of the lumen because of edema, and a scalloped margin of the bowel wall resembling thumb prints or pseudodiverticula caused by intramural hematomas. It is difficult to distinguish ischemic colitis from regional enteritis, but the former does not cause fistula formation.

Ischemic colitis is also observed in women taking oral contraceptives. This is of diagnostic importance. The course is typical with rapid disappearance of symptoms in a matter of days [40, 41, 53, 54, 56, 127, 178, 191, 204].

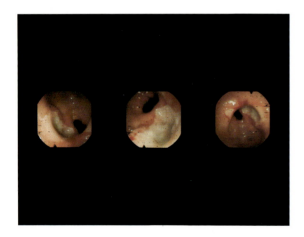

FIGURE 390
Ischemic colitis in the upper portion of the descending colon superficial and deep punched-out ulcers in the red, edematous mucosa.

References

[1] AKOVBIANTZ, A., AEBERHARD, P., ARMA, S.: Kolondivertikulose – Divertikulitis. Schweiz. Rundschau Med. (Praxis) *57*, 375 (1968).

[2] ALEXANDER-WILLIAMS, J., BUCHMANN, P.: Perianale Komplikationen beim Morbus Crohn. In: Entzündliche Erkrankungen des Dickdarms, 296–306. Ed. R. Ottenjann, H. Fahrländer, Berlin, Heidelberg, New York, Tokio: Springer (1983).

[3] ALLEGRA, G.: Le mélanome anorectale. Ann. de Gastroentérologie et d'Hép. *21,* 6, 365–369 (1985).

[4] AMBROSE, N.S., MORRIS, D., ALEXANDER-WILLIAMS, J., KEIGHLEY, M.R.: A randomized trial of photocoagulation or injection sclerotherapy for the treatment of first and second degree hemorrhoids. Dis. Colon Rectum *28,* 4, 238–240 (1985).

[5] AMGWERD, R.F.: Das Hämorrhoidalleiden, Wann sind welche Verfahren indiziert? DIA – GM, *18,* 29 (1984).

[6] BARBER, G.B. et al.: Refractory Distal Ulcerative Colitis Responsive to 5-Aminosalicylate Enemas. Am. J. Gastroenterol. *80,* 612–614 (1985).

[7] BARRON, J.: Office ligation of internal hemorrhoids. Amer. J. Surg. *105,* 563 (1963).

[8] BAUMGARTNER, R.: Behandlung innerer Hämorrhoiden mit elastischen Ligaturen. Schweiz. med. Wschr. *100,* 1249 (1970).

[9] BENSAUDE, R.: Rectoscopie, sigmoidoscopie. Masson, Paris (1956).

[10] BENSAUDE, A.: Les hémorroïdes et affections courantes de la région anale. Libr. Maloine S.A., Paris (1967).

[11] BENSAUDE, A.: Zur Bedeutung der portalen Drucksteigerung bei der Ätiopathogenese der Hämorrhoiden. Colo-Proctology *6,* 394–396 (1981).

[12] BERCHTOLD, R.: Maligne Rektum- und Analtumoren, Gastroent. Fortbildungsk. Praxis. Vol. *3,* 99–104, Karger, Basel (1973).

[13] BERNIER, J.-J.: Gastroentérologie 2. Flammarion méd. sciences Paris (1984).

[14] BESSON, A., DELACRETAZ, F.: Pneumatose, Kystique intestinale. Schweiz. Rundschau Med. (Praxis) *73,* Nr. 46, 1407–1415 (1984).

[15] BIGARD, M.: Ulceration tuberculeuse perianale isolée. Presse Méd. *14,* (4), 231 (1985).

[16] BILLEBAND, T., MOLKON, J.-M., HOURY, S., LACAINE, F. et HUQUIER, M.: La radiothérapie dans les adénocarcinomes du rectum. Gastroenterol. Clin. Biol. *9,* 437–443 (1985).

[17] BLASER, M.J., RELLER, L.R.: Campylobacter enteritis. N. Engl. J. Med. *305,* 1444–1452 (1981).

[18] BLOND, K., HOFF, H.: Das Hämorrhoidalleiden. Deuticke, Leipzig/Wien (1936).

[19] BOEHM, C., SCHMID, A.H., WENZEL, M.: Das Hämorrhoidalleiden. Schattauer, Stuttgart (1967).

[20] BOGNEL, J.C.: Polypes familiales diffuses. Ann. de Gastroentérologie et d'Hépatologie *21,* 6, 347–350 (1985).

[21] BOULIS WASSIF, S., CASPERS, R.J.L.: Die Therapie des analen Karzinoms. Colo-Proctology *4,* 228–231 (1983).

[22] LE BOURGEOIS, P.C., POYNARD, T., MODAI, J., MARCHE, C., AVRIL, M.F., CHAPUT, J.C.: Ulceration peri-anale. Ne pas oublier la tuberculose. Presse Méd. *13* (41), 2507–2509 (1984).

[23] BRUEHL, W.: Kausale Behandlung des Hämorrhoidalleiden. Colo-Proctology 5, Nr. *1,* 38 (1983).

[24] BUCHMANN, P., WETERMAN, I.T.: Der perianale Morbus Crohn. Colo-Proctology *2,* 77–81 (1981).

[25] BUCHMANN, P.: Lehrbuch der Proktologie. Huber, Bern (1988).

[26] BUCHMANN, P.: Spezielle Fisteln und Analabszesse. Schweiz. Med. Rundsch. (Praxis) *74* (35), 902–904 (1985).

[27] BUCHMANN, P.: Therapie der Analkomplikation des Morbus Crohn. Schweiz. Rundschau Med. (Praxis) *75,* 11, 291–294 (1986).

[28] BURKITT, D.P.: Diet and its Relation to Hemorrhoids. Colo-Proctology *5,* 315–316 (1980).

[29] BUSSY, H.J.R.: Gastrointestinal polyposis syndromes in Recent Advances in Histopathology ed. by Antony P.P., Macsween R.N.M., Nr. *12*, 169–177 (1984).

[30] CAMPIERI, M. et al.: Treatment of ulcerative Colitis with highdose 5-Aminosalicyl acid enemas. Lancet, 8241 *II*, 270–271 (1981).

[31] CATALAN, F.: Les maladies sexuellement transmissibles en proctologie. Schweiz. Rundschau Med. (Praxis) *72*, Nr. 28, 953–959 (1983).

[32] CLEMENÇON, G.: Pneumatosis cystoides intestini, Gastroent. Fortbildungsk. Praxis. Vol. *3*, 116–125, Karger, Basel (1973).

[33] COPÉ, R.: Atlas de la Maladie hémorroïdaire. Ed. Louis Pariente, Paris (1983).

[34] COTTIER, H.: Pathogenese. Springer Verlag Berlin, Heidelberg, New York, Tokio (1980).

[35] COTTIER, H., GOLAY, L., MANGOLD, R.: Pathogenese und Klinik der Pneumatosis cystoides des Dickdarms. Gastroenterologia, Basel *92*, 224 (1959).

[36] COTTON, P.B., WILLIAMS, CH.B.: Practical Gastrointestinal Endoscopy. Blackwell scientific Publications, Oxford, London (1980).

[37] CROHN, B.B., YARNIS, H., CROHN, E.B., WALTER, R.I., GABRILOVE, L.J.: Ulcerative colitis and pregnancy. Gastroenterology *30*, 391 (1956).

[38] CROHN, B.B., GINZBURG, L., OPPENHEIMER, G.D.: Regional Ileitis, A Pathologic and Clinical Entity. JAMA *99*, 1323–1329 (1932).

[39] CRONKHITE, L.E., CANADA, W.J.: Generalized gastrointestinal polyposis. New Engl. J. Med. *252*, 1011 (1955).

[40] CYNN, W.S., RICKERT, R.R.: Ischemic proctosigmoiditis. Dis. Col. + Rect. *16*, 537 (1973).

[41] DE LOS RIOS MAGRINA, E.: Atlas de Colo-Proctologie. MEDSI, Paris (1981).

[42] DENIS, J. et al.: Laser CO_2 en proctologie: Mythes et Réalités à propos de 587 interventions-Laser, Gastroentérologie clinique et Biologique, Masson, Paris, Vol. *8*, No. 2bis, 161A (1984).

[43] DETRANO, S.J.: Die Prinzipien der Kryobiologie in der Kryochirurgie. Colo-Proctology *6*, 398–399 (1980).

[44] DEUCHER, F., NÖTHIGER, F.: Der transanale Eingriff beim Rektumkarzinom. Chirurg *49*, 260–264 (1978).

[45] DEVLIN, M.B. et al.: Klysma: Ein altes Mittel – modern angewendet. Proktologie *1*, 43–45 (1979).

[46] DEW, M.J.: An oral Preparation to release drugs in the Human Colon. Brit. J. clin. Pharmac. *14*, 405–408 (1982).

[47] DIETRICH, K.F.: Proktologie für die Praxis. Lehmanns Verl., München (1969).

[48] DITTRICH, H.: Zur Geschichte der gastroenterologischen Endoskopie. Wien. Klin. Wschr., im Druck.

[49] DRITZ, S.K., GOLDSMITH, R.S.: Sexually transmissible protozoal bacterial and viral enteric infections. Comp. Ther. *6*, 34–40 (1980).

[50] DUHAMEL, J.: Proctologie aux divers âges. Flammarion méd. sciences Paris (1972).

[51] DUEHRSEN, K., KIRCH, W., BRITTINGER, G., OHNHAUS, E., REINWEIN, D.: Das Behçet Syndrom. Schweiz. med. Wschr. *114*, 1058–1068 (1984).

[52] EFSTRADIATIS, N., FLEISCHER, K., DROESZUS, J.-N.: Pneumatosis cystoides intestinalis bei Dolicho-Sigma mit funktionellen Beschwerden. Z. Gastroenterologie *20*, 631–637 (1982).

[53] EGGER, G., KELLOCK, T.D.: Akute regionäre Kolitis – ischämische Kolitis. Schweiz. med. Wschr. *100*, 1264 (1970).

[54] EGGER, G., HAERTEL, M., HALTER, F., LAISSUE, J.: Die nicht gangränöse ischämische Colitis: Klinik und radiologische Diagnostik. Röfo, *115*, 432 (1971).

[55] EGGER, G., WITZEL, L.: Strahlenschäden des Gastrointestinaltraktes. Fortschritte der Medizin, Bd. *11*, 834 (1974).

[56] EGGER, G., MANGOLD, R.: Ischaemic colitis and contraceptives. Acta hepatogastroent. *21*, 221 (1974).

[57] EHSANULLAH, M., FILIPE, M., GAZZARD, B.: Morphological and mucus secretion criteria for different diagnosis of solitary ulcer syndrome and non-specific proctitis. J. clin. Path. *35*, 26–30 (1982).

[58] EHSANULLAH, M., ISAACS, A., ISABELFILIPE, M., GAZZARD, B.G.: Tuberculosis presenting as inflammatory bowel disease. Report of two cases. Dis. Colon Rectum, 134–136 (1984).

[59] EICHMANN, A.: Sexuell übertragbare Krankheiten nach Reisen in tropische Länder. Therapeutische Umschau, 42, Heft *11*, 805–811 (1985).

[60] EICHMANN, A.: Sexuell übertragbare Krankheiten in der perianalen und in der perinealen Region. Schweiz. Rundschau Med. (Praxis) *74,* Nr. 35, 919–922 (1985).

[61] EIGLER, F.W. u. Mitarb.: Therapie des Analkarzinoms. Ein komb. chir.-radiologisches Konzept. Münch. med. Wschr. 124, Nr. *32/33,* 706–720 (1982).

[62] ELBERG, J.J.: Oxygen therapie for pneumatosis coli. Acta chir. Scand. 151, 399–400 (1985).

[63] EWE, K.: Dickdarm: In Gastro-Enterologie, herausgegeben von Clodi, P.H. 104–136. Springer Verlag Berlin, Heidelberg, New York, Tokio (1985).

[64] EWE, K., OTTO, P.: Atlas der Rektoskopie und Koloskopie. Springer, Berlin (1984).

[65] FAHRLAENDER, H.: Klinik, Ätiologie und Therapie der pseudomembranösen Kolitis. Schweiz. Rundschau Med. (Praxis) *71,* 92–97 (1982).

[66] FAHRLAENDER, H.: Epidemiologie, Pathogenese, Verlauf und Folgen der Crohnschen Erkrankung. Schweiz. med. Wschr. *115,* Suppl. 19, 21–29 (1985).

[67] FLUCKER, J.L.: Homosexually Transmitted Infections. Schweiz. Rundschau Med. (Praxis) 72, Nr. *30,* 997–999 (1983).

[68] FRANK, W., WANNER, G., KOEST, H.-P.: Die Kryptoglanduläre Entzündung: Untersuchung zur Fistelentstehung, Colo-Proctology *1,* 7–12 (1985).

[69] FREEMANN, J.G. et al.: Sulphasalazine and Spermatogenesis. Digestion *23,* 68–71 (1982).

[70] FRUEHMORGEN, P., DEMLING, P.: Complications of diagnostic and therapeutic coloscopy in Federal Republic of Germany. Results of an inquiry. Endoscopy *11,* 146 (1979).

[71] GARDNER, E.J., RICHARD, R.C.: Multiple cutaneous and subcutaneous lesions obscurring simultaneously with hereditary polyposis and osteomatosis. Amer. J. hum. genet. *5,* 139–147 (1953).

[72] GARREN VAN, H.: Schneiden und Koagulieren mit hochfrequenten Strömen. Proktologie *3,* 190–191 (1980).

[73] GEBBERS, J.-O., ALTERMATT, H.J., LAISSUE, J.-A.: Vor- und Frühstadien des kolorektalen Karzinoms. Schweiz. Rundschau Med. (Praxis) 79, Nr. *5,* 89–100 (1990).

[74] GEBBERS, J.-O., LAISSUE, J.-A.: Pathologie der Analtumoren. Schweiz. Rundschau Med. (Praxis) 73, Nr. *27,* 847–862 (1984).

[75] GEBOES, K. et al.: Acute Colitis due to Campylobacter Infect. Colo-Proctology *5,* 292–295 (1980).

[76] GELFAND, M.D., TEPPER, M., KATZ, L.A. et al.: Acute irradiation proctitis in man. Gastroenterology *54,* 401 (1968).

[77] GEMSENJAEGER, E.: Hämorrhoiden. Eine Übersicht über altes und neues Wissen. Schweiz. Rundschau Med. (Praxis) 72, Nr. *25,* 862–870 (1983).

[78] GEMSENJAEGER, E.: Lokale Exzision bei Rektumkarzinom. Schweiz. Rundschau Med. (Praxis) 76, Nr. *20,* 551–557 (1987).

[79] GIRONA, J.: Submuköse Hämorrhoidektomie nach Parks. Colo-Proctology *2,* 125–127 (1981).

[80] GLOOR, F.: Die morphologische Differentialdiagnose der chronischen, unspezifischen, ulzerösen Kolitis. Schweiz. med. Wschr. 101, Nr. *20,* 690–697 (1971).

[81] GLOOR, F.: Die nicht klassifizierbaren ulzerösen Kolitiden. Schweiz. med. Wschr. *111,* 779–783 (1981).

[82] GLOOR, F.: Was bringt die Histologie in der Differentialdiagnose anorektaler Erkrankungen? Swiss Med 7, Nr. *1a,* 33–36 (1985).

[83] GOLIGHER, J.C.: Surgery of the Anus, Rectum and Colon. Baillère Tindal, London (1975).

[84] GREANY, M.G., IRVIN, CH.M.: Criteria of the selection of rectal cancers for local treatment. Dis. Col. Rect. *20,* 463 (1977).

[85] GYR, K.: Parasitäre Colitis. Schweiz. Rundschau Med. (Praxis) 73, Nr. *34,* 1033–1036 (1984).

[86] HAAS, D.: Rektosigmoidnekrose nach Hämorrhoidenverödung. Helf. chir. Acta, *43,* 591–592 (1976).

[87] HABAL, F.M., GREENBERG, G.R.: Oral 5-ASA in the treatment of ulcerative colitis. Gastroenterology Vol. 88, Nr. *5,* Pat 2 (1983).

[88] HAECKI, W.H.: Strahlenproktokolitis, die Kehrseite der Medaille. Schweiz. Rundschau Med. (Praxis) 73, Nr. *35,* 1065–1069 (1984).

[89] HAFTER, E.: Praktische Gastroenterologie. Thieme, Stuttgart (1978). (Neuaufl. 1987).

[90] HALLER, O., ZBINDEN, R.: Herpes genitalis. Therapeutische Umschau 42, Heft *11,* 793–797 (1985).

[91] HALLER VON, A.: Primae lineae physiologiae. Ap. Viduam Ab Vandenhoeck, Acad. Bibl. Gottingae, S. 486 (MDCCLI).

[92] HALTER, F., NEIGER, A.: Prokto-, Rekto- und Sigmoidoskopie. In Gastroenterologische Endoskopie von Ottenjann, R., Classen, M., Enke Verl. Stuttgart, 216–242 (1979).

[93] HANSEN, H., STELZNER, F.: Proktologie, Springer, Berlin (1981).

[94] HANSEN, H.H.: Neue Aspekte zur Pathogenese und Therapie des Hämorrhoidalleidens. Dtsch. med. Wschr. 102, 1244–1248 (1977).

[95] HEER, M.: Ungewöhnliche Formen chronisch entzündlicher Dickdarmerkrankungen. Schweiz. Rundschau Med. (Praxis) 75, 11, 295–302 (1986).

[96] HEER, M., SALFINGER, M., KEHL, O., MUENCH, R., BUEHLER, H., STAMM, B., HANY, A., AMMANN, R.: Die primäre Kolontuberkulose. Schweiz. med. Wschr. 115, 349–353 (1985).

[97] HEINKEL, K., ELSTER, K., HENNING, N., LANDGRAF, J.: Die Saugprobeexzision aus dem Rektum. Klin. Wschr. 38, 578 (1960).

[98] HERMAUCK, P.: Zur Differentialdiagnose segmentärer ulzeröser Kolonveränderungen. Verh. Dtsch. Ges. Path. 54, 381 (1970).

[99] HUGES, E.P., VEIDENHEIMER, M.C., CORMAN, M.L. et al.: Electrocoagulation of rectal cancer. Dis. Colon Rectum 25, 215–218 (1982).

[100] JUERGEN, T., GROITL, H., HAGER, T.: Komplikationen bei endoskopischen Untersuchungen des Dickdarmes. Proktologie 3, 185–189 (1980).

[101] KEIGHLEY, M.R.B.: Randomisierte Studie zum Vergleich von Photokoagulation und Gummiringligatur bei der Behandlung von Hämorrhoiden. Colo-Proctology 2, 132–134 (1982).

[102] KEIGHLEY, M.R.B.: Pseudomembranous Colitis. Schweiz. Rundschau Med. (Praxis) 71, 98–106 (1982).

[103] KIEFHABER, P., KIEFHABER, K., HUBER, F., GUTHY, E., NATH, G.: The application of the infraredcoagulators in gastroenterology and surgery. Optoelektronik in der Medizin. Vortrag des 6. Internationalen Kongresses Laser 1983. Herausgeber W. Waidlizh. S. 75. Springer Verlag, Berlin, Heidelberg, New York, Tokio (1984).

[104] KLOSTERMANN, G.F.: Pigmentfleckenpolypose (Thieme, Stuttgart, 1960).

[105] KLOTZ, U., MAIER, K.E.: Chronisch-entzündliche Darmerkrankungen. Therapiewoche 35, 3895–3903 (1985).

[106] KRAUSE, H.: Hautmykosen. DIA – GM 17, 26–34 (1985).

[107] KUTZNER, J. et al.: Strahlenproktitis als Folge onkologischer Radiotherapie. Proktologie 3, 14–19 (1979).

[108] LANG, G.: Pneumatosis coli. Schweiz. Rundschau Med. (Praxis) 73, Nr. 35, 1061–1064, (1984).

[109] LEHNER, T.: Rezidivierende Mundgeschwüre und Behçet-Syndrom. Hexagon «Roche» 11, Nr. 1, 7–12 (1983).

[110] LEICESTER, R.J., NICHOLS, R.J., MANN, C.V.: Infrared coagulation: a new treatment for hemorrhoids. Dis Colon Rectum 24, 602 (1981).

[111] LEICESTER, R.J., NICHOLS, R.J., MANN, C.V.: Vergleichende Studie über Infrarot-Koagulation und konventionelle Methoden in der Hämorrhoiden-Therapie. Colo-Proctologie 5, 313–315 (1981).

[112] LEDERBOGEN, K.: Rektoskopie, Sigmoidoskopie, Koloskopie. G. Thieme, Stuttgart (1984).

[113] LENTINI, J.: Temas de Coloproctologia. Ed. Fontalba, Barcelona (1982).

[114] LENTINI, J., TAURE, C., LEVERONI, J.: Venerische Erkrankung des Anus und Rektums. Proktologie 3, 196–201 (1980).

[115] LENTINI, I., TAURE, D., LEVORINI, J.: Nouvelles considérations sur la condylomatose anale. Gastroentérologie Clinique et Biologique, 10, 2, 57 A (1986).

[116] LESKY, E.: Die Wiener medizinische Schule im 19. Jahrhundert. Studien zur Geschichte der Universität Wien, Vol. VI. Böhlaus Nachf., Graz-Köln (1965).

[117] LESKY, E.: Die Wiener Experimente mit dem Lichtleiter Bozzinis (1806/1807). Clio Medica, Vol. 5, 327–350 (1970) (Pergamon Press, Oxford).

[118] LIEBESKIND, M., MALBRAN, J., AGARD, D., PANNETTER, C., LECOUILLARED, G., IVANOVIC, A.: Manifestations anorectales des maladies sexuellements transmissibles. Sarcome de Kaposi. Ann. Gastroentérol.-Hépatol. 20, 5, 265–270 (1984).

[119] LEWIS, I.M. et al.: Cryosurgical Hemorrhoidectomy. Diseases of the Colon + Rectum. Vol. 12, No. 5, 371 (1969).

[120] LORD, P.H.: A new regime of the treatment of hemorrhoids. Proc. roy. Soc. Med. *61,* 935 (1968).

[121] LORENZ, R., GULOTTA, U., BECKER, K., BOTTERMANN, P., VOGEL, G.E., CLASSEN, M.: Neue Beobachtungen bei einem Fall von Cronkhite-Canada-Syndrom. Z. Gastroenterologie *24,* 85–92 (1986).

[122] LURZ, K.H.: Gummibandligatur von Hämorrhoiden mit neuer Aspirationstechnik. Proktologie *1,* 59–60 (1980).

[123] MADIGAN, M.R., MORSON, B.C.: Solitary ulcer of the rectum. Gut *10,* 871 (1969).

[124] MANN, G.: Der Frankfurter Lichtleiter. Neues über Philipp Bozzini und sein Endoskop. Medizin historisches Journal, Bd. *8,* 105–130 (1973) (Georg Olms Verlag, Hildesheim).

[125] MARKOWITZ, J., DAUM, F., AIGES, H., KAHN, E., SILVERBERG, M., FISHER, St.E.: Perianal Disease in Children and Adolescents with Crohn's Disease. Gastroenetrol. *86,* 829–833 (1984).

[126] MARKS, G.: Histopathologische Wirkung der Infrarotkoagulation. Colo-Proctology *3,* 183–184 (1981).

[127] MARSTON, A., PHEILS, M.-T., THOMAS, L., MORSON, B.C.: Ischaemic colitis. Gut *7,* 1 (1966).

[128] MARTI, M.-C.: Les fissures anales. Schweiz. Rundschau Med. (Praxis) 65, Nr. *45,* 1398–1403 (1976).

[129] MARTI, M.-C.: Les fistules anales. Schweiz. Rundschau Med. (Praxis) 74, Nr. *35,* 898–901 (1985).

[130] MARTI, M.-C., CEREDA, J.M.: Primärtuberkulose des Anus. Beschreibung zweier Fälle. Proktologie *2,* 151–152 (1980).

[131] MARTI, M.-C., NOETHIGER, F.: Incontinence anale et chirurgie de renforcement de l'appareil sphincterien. Schweiz. Rundschau Med. (Praxis) *70,* 679–687 (1981).

[132] MARTI, M.-C., GIVEL, J.-C.: Surgery of Anorectal Diseases. Springer, Berlin (1990).

[133] MASON, A.: Malignant tumors of the rectum. Local excision. Clin. Gastroenterol. *4,* 582 (1975).

[134] MENTHA, J., NEIGER, A., MANGOLD, R.: Entzündungen des Anus und Hämorrhoiden. Praxis *50,* 751 (1961).

[135] MEYER, J.Chr., EICHMANN, A.: Serodiagnostik und Therapie der Syphilis. Therapeutische Umschau, Vol. *42,* 773–780 (1985).

[136] MILES, R.P.M.: Lymphogranuloma of anorectum. Proc. Roy. Soc. Med. *55,* 873 (1962).

[137] MILLIGAN, E.T.C., MORGAN, C.N., JONES, L.E., OFFICER, R.: Surgical anatomy of the anal canal, and the operative treatment of hemorrhoids. Lancet *2,* 1119–1124 (1937).

[138] MOHR, W.: Amöbiasis. Hexagon «Roche» 1, 11–17 (1987).

[139] MONTORSI, W.: Le emorroidi e il loro tratamento. Arch. Soc. Ital. di chir. Masson, Paris (1984).

[140] MORSON, B.C.: The muscle abnormality in the diverticular disease of the colon. Proc. roy. Soc. Med. *56,* 22 (1963).

[141] MORSON, B.C.: The technique and interpretation of rectal biopsy in inflammatory bowel disease. Pathol. Annu. *9,* 205 (1974).

[142] MÜNCH, R., BÜHLER, H.: Morbus Crohn und Colitis ulcerosa: Internistische Aspekte der Diagnose und der Therapie. Schweiz. Rundschau Med. (Praxis) 75, *11,* 277–282 (1986).

[143] MULLER, C.A.: Internal Hemorrhoidectomy by Rubber Band Ligation. Colo-Proctology *5,* 317–319 (1980).

[144] MULLER, C.A.: Hémorroïdectomie interne par ligatures élastiques. Indications, limites. Schweiz. Rundschau Med. (Praxis) *71,* 196–198 (1982).

[145] MULLER, G.: Die enteralen Fisteln beim Morbus Crohn. Schweiz. Rundschau Med. (Praxis) 73, Nr. *48,* 1477–1587 (1984).

[146] MUSEK, J.: Kryochirurgie in der Behandlung inoperabler Tumoren von Rektum und Anus. Colo-Proctology *1,* 47–48 (1983).

[147] NATH, G.: Physikalische Grundlagen des neuen Prinzips der Infrarot-Koagulation in der Medizin. Colo-Proctology *6,* 379–381 (1981).

[148] NEIGER, A.: Rektoskopische Verlaufskontrolle des röntgenkontaktbestrahlten Rektumkarzinoms. Z. Gastroent. Verh. bd. *IV* (1970).

[149] NEIGER, A.: Die Sigmoidoskopie mit flexiblen Instrumenten in der ambulanten Praxis. Z. Gastroenterologie *10,* 421–424 + 634–635 (1972) + Schweiz. med. Wschr. *102,* 1022–1024 (1972).

[150] NEIGER, A.: Die Behandlung des einfachen Hämorrhoidalleidens. Therapeutische Umschau *29,* 26–30 (1972).

158

[151] NEIGER, A.: Komplikationen bei der Fibersigmoidoskopie. Z. Gastroenterologie *12,* 47 (1974).

[152] NEIGER, A.: Die diffuse Polypose des Dickdarmes. Z. Gastroenterologie *5,* 541–542 (1975).

[153] NEIGER, A.: Erfahrungen mit Doxiproct® und Doxiproct Plus® Suppositorien bei der Behandlung des Hämorrhoidalleidens. Folia Angiologica *23,* 433–435 (1975).

[154] NEIGER, A.: Proctitis terminalis simplex. Z. Gastroenterology *14,* 694 (1976).

[155] NEIGER, A.: Erfahrungen mit dem Strangler, einem Ligaturanoskop. Z. Gastroenterologie *15,* 602–603 (1977).

[156] NEIGER, A.: Proktologische Sprechstunde. I–IV Analblutungen, Untersuchungsgang, Beh., Hexagon «Roche» *5,* Nr. *2,* 3, 4, 6–7 (1977).

[157] NEIGER, A.: Le traitement sclérosant des hémorrhoides par coagulation à l'infrarouge. Annales Gastr. et Hépat. *13,* 7, 701–705 (1977).

[158] NEIGER, A.: Hämorrhoiden: Erkennung und heutige Behandlungsmöglichkeiten. Schw. Med. Wschr. *108,* 500 (1978).

[159] NEIGER, A.: Das kolorektale Karzinom. Ärztliche Praxis *31,* 1466–1467 (1979).

[160] NEIGER, A.: Entzündungen im Analbereich. Dtsch. Ärzteblatt 76, Heft *41,* 2639–2643 (1979).

[161] NEIGER, A.: Pathogenese, Klinik und konservative Therapie des Hämorrhoidalleidens. Schweiz. med. Wschr. *110,* 1387–1290 (1980).

[162] NEIGER, A.: Analtumoren. Hexagon «Roche» 9, Nr. *4,* 12–17 (1981).

[163] NEIGER, A.: Analfissuren. Hexagon «Roche» 9, Nr. *6,* 16 (1981) + Urologe (B) 22, 201–205 (1982).

[164] NEIGER, A.: Hämorrhoiden-Verödungsbehandlung durch Infrarotkoagulation. Schweiz. Rundschau Med. (Praxis) *71,* 171–176 (1982).

[165] NEIGER, A.: Konservative Behandlung des Hämorrhoidalleidens. Dtsch. Med. Wschr. 107, Nr. *15,* 589–590 (1982).

[166] NEIGER, A.: Diagnose, Differentialdiagnose und Therapie entzündlicher und nicht entzündlicher Hämorrhoidalerkrankungen in der Praxis. Internist. prax. *23,* 37–63 (1983).

[167] NEIGER, A.: Klinik und Lokalbefund der Analtumoren. Schweiz. Rundschau Med. (Praxis) 73, Nr. *27,* 863–865 (1984).

[168] NEIGER, A.: Pruritus ani und Proktalgia nocturna. Swiss med. *7,* 37–38 (1985).

[169] NEIGER, A.: Morbus Crohn – anale und ·perianale Manifestationen. Hexagon «Roche» 13, Nr. *1,* 9–12, Suppl. (1985).

[170] NEIGER, A., MORITZ, K., KIEFHABER, P.: Hämorrhoiden-Verödungsbehandlung durch Infrarotkoagulation. In Fortschritte der gastroenterologischen Endoskopie (H. Henning) Bd. 9, *102* (1977) Verl. Gerh. Witzstrock, Baden-Baden.

[171] NICHOLS, J., GLASS, R.: Coloproctology. Springer Verlag, Berlin, Heidelberg, New York, Tokio (1985).

[172] NOETHIGER, F.: Indikationen und Grenzen der chirurgischen Behandlung von Hämorrhoiden. Schweiz. Rundschau Med. (Praxis) 71, Nr. *5,* 193–195 (1982).

[173] NOETHIGER, F.: Lokale, peranale Tumorexzision. Helv. chir. Acta *50,* 623–627 (1983).

[174] NOETHIGER, F.: Technique and results of peranal excision of rectal malignoma. Helv. chir. Acta *52,* 325–327 (1985).

[175] NOETHIGER, F.: Rektumprolaps. Schweiz. Rundschau Med. (Praxis), (1986).

[176] NOETHIGER, F., HASSLER, H.: Traitement chirurgical de la rectocolite hémorragique. Méd. et Hyg. *42,* 2830–2838 (1984).

[177] OTTENJANN, P.: Divertikulose und Divertikulitis des Dickdarmes. Münch. med. Wschr. *116,* 1069 (1974).

[178] OTTENJANN, P.: Atlas der Koloileoskopie. Ferd. Enke Stuttgart, 1–22 (1980).

[179] OTTENJANN, P., FAHRLAENDER, H.: Entzündliche Erkrankungen des Dickdarmes. Springer, Berlin (1983).

[180] OTTO, P.: Das Hämorrhoidalleiden. Z. Hautkr. 50 (8), 315–324 (1975) Grosse Verl.

[181] OTTO, P.: Erfahrungen mit der Infrarot-Koagulation in der Behandlung des Hämorrhoidalleidens. Colo-Proctology 2, 129–131 (1982).

[182] OTTO, P., WETTENGEL, R.: Blutgasanalysen des Hämorrhoidalblutes. Ein Beitrag zur Diskussion über eine arterielle oder venöse Versorgung des Corpus cavernosum recti. Phlebol. u. Proktol. *1,* 254 (1972).

[183] OWEN, W.F. Jr.: Medical problems of the homosexual adolescent. J. Adolesc. Health Care *6* (4), 278–285 (1985).

[184] PAPILLON, J. et coll.: Place de la radiothérapie dans le traitement du cancer de l'anus au début. Arch. Mal. App. Dig. *57,* 57–73 (1968).

[185] PAPILLON, J.: Place de la radiothérapie à visée curative dans le traitement des adenocarcinomes du rectum et des carcinomes malpighiens du canal anal. Med Chir Dig *10,* 239–242 (1981).

[186] PAPILLON, J.: Rectal and anal cancers. Springer Verlag, New York, 126–175 (1982).

[187] PAPILLON, J. et al.: A new approach to the management of epidermoid carcinoma of the anal canal. Cancer *56,* 1830–1837 (1983).

[188] PAPILLON, J.: Nouvelles perspectives dans le traitement conservateur du cancer du rectum. Méd. Chir. Dig. *14,* 507–510 (1985).

[189] PARKS, A.G.: The surgical treatment of hemorrhoids. Brit. J. Surg. *43,* 337 (1956).

[190] PARKS, A.G., GORDON, P.H., HARDCASTLE, J.G.: A classification of fistula-in-ano. Br. J. Surg. *63,* -R (1976).

[191] PARKS, T.G.: Ischämische Kolonerkrankungen. Colo-Proctologie *4,* 213–218 (1980).

[192] PARKS, T.G.: Pathogenese, Diagnose und Therapie des solitären Rektumulkus. Colo-Proctology *4,* 236–238 (1983).

[193] PARKS, T.G.: Die Pathophysiologie der unkomplizierten Kolondivertikulose. Colo-Proctology *1,* 41–44 (1983).

[194] PARNAUD, E., GUNTZ, M., BERNARD, A., CHOME, J.: Anatomie normale macroscopique et microscopique du réseau vasculaire hémorroïdal. Arch. Fr. Mal. App. Dig. *65,* 500–514 (1976).

[195] PARNAUD, E., GUNTZ, M., BIDART, J.M., BERNARD, A., CHOME, J.: Considération sur la vascularisation normale de la sousmuqueuse anale. Incidences sur la nature de la maladie hémorroïdaire. Rev. Proct. *1,* 44 (1981).

[196] PARNAUD, E., BAUER, P.: Localisations digestives des maladies sexuellement transmissibles chez l'homosexuel male. Presse Med. *14* (23), 1282–1286 (1985).

[197] PARTURIER-ALBOT, M.: Diagnostic précoce des tumeurs du rectum et leurs traitements (Contactthérapie et radiochirurgie). In Albot, G., Poilleux, F.: Intestin grêle côlonrectum. Actualités hépato-gastroentérol. Hôtel-Dieu 1955, p. 281, Masson, Paris (1956).

[198] PARTURIER-ALBOT, M.: Les aspects morphologiques du cancer de l'anus. Leurs correspondances évolutives et leurs possibilités thérapeutiques (Formes de début). Arch. Mal. App. dig. *49,* 7/8bis: 2 (1960).

[199] PARTURIER-ALBOT, M.: Die Röntgenkontaktbestrahlung des Frühkarzinoms des Anus und des Rektums, Gastroent. Fortbildungsk. Praxis, Vol. *3,* 105–115, Karger, Basel (1973).

[200] PARTURIER-ALBOT, M., BENSAUDE, A., REY, M.: Aspects particulières de certains tumeurs anales ou maladie de Bowen à localisation anale. Gaz. Méd. France 75, *30* (1968).

[201] PARTURIER-ALBOT, M., PREVOST, A.G., ALBOT, G., BOLGERT, M.: Les carcinomes multicentriques de la région anorectale. Ann. Gastro-entérol. Hépatol. 18, *4,* 227–235 (1982).

[202] PARTURIER-ALBOT, M., ALBOT, G.: Le carcinom «de nowo» ou carcinom d'emblée du rectum. Fréquense et éléments de diagnostic. Ann. de Gastroentérologie et d'Hépatologie. 21, *4,* 231–237 (1985).

[203] PEYER DE, R.: Colopathies aux laxatifs. Schweiz. Rundschau Med. (Praxis) 73, Nr. *34,* 1037–1039 (1984).

[204] PIMPL, W., UMLAUFT, M.: Ischämische Kolitis nach kardiogenem Schock. Colo-Proctology *1,* 15–18 (1983).

[205] PIPARD, G.: Radiothérapie des cancers de l'anus. Schweiz. Rundschau Med. (Praxis) 73, Nr. *28,* 888–893 (1984).

[206] POPPEL VAN, H.P., CHRISTIAENS, M.R.: Die anale Aktinomykose. Colo-Proctology *5,* 322–326 (1981).

[207] PRADEL, E.: Maladie de Paget et de Bowen de l'anus. Rev. Proct. *1,* 11–26 (1982).

[208] PRADEL, E., BARIERA, E., JUILLARD, F., TERRIS, G.: Anorektale Ulzera homosexueller Genese. Colo-Proctology *1,* 47–52 (1985).

[209] PREVOST, A.-G., LANGERON, P., MALBEZIN, E.: Polypose rectocolique diffuse. Etude d'une observation familiale. J. Sci. méd. Lille *89,* 51 (1971).

[210] PREVOST, A.-G.: Die diffuse Polypose des Rektums. Gastroent. Fortbildungsk. Vol. *3,* 92–98, Karger, Basel (1973).

[211] PRICE, A.B., DAY, D.W.: Pseudomembranous and infective colitis. In Recent Advances in Histopathology, Ed. by Antony, P.P. Maesween, R.N.M., Nr. *11,* 99–117 (1981), Curchill Livingstone, Edinburgh, London.

[212] QUINN, T.C., GOODELL, S.E., MKRTICHIAN, E., SCHUFFLER, M.D., WANG, S.P., STAMM, W.E., HOLMES, K.K.: Chlamydia trachomatis proctitis. N. Engl. J. Med. *305*, 195 (1981).

[213] RAIMBERT, P. et al.: Photocoagulation infrarouge en proctologie: premiers résultats. Rev. Proct. *3*, 199–205 (1981).

[214] RAUSIS, C., ARNOLD, J.: Indications et limites de la cryochirurgie des hémorroïdes. Schweiz. Rundschau Med. (Praxis) *71*, 181–185 (1982).

[215] RAUSIS, C.: Chirurgie des hémorroïdes avec laser CO_2. Schweiz. Rundschau Med. (Praxis) *71*, 177–180 (1982).

[216] RENE, E.: Les lésions recto-coliques du Sida. Réunion soc. nat. franc. de proctologie, Paris 16.11.1985.

[217] RICK, M., HALTER, F., STIRNEMANN, H.: Das solitäre Rektalulkus. Schweiz. med. Wschr. *101*, 758 (1971).

[218] RICK, M., HALTER, F.: Das solitäre Rektumulkus. Gastroent. Fortbildungsk. Praxis, Vol. *3*, 65–70, Karger, Basel (1973).

[219] RODIER, B., FOISSY, P., ESPINOZA, P.: Sténose rectale avec fistule anale localisation basse d'une tuberculose colique. Gastroentérologie Clinique et Biologique *10*, 2, 59A (1986).

[220] ROSCHKE, W.: Zur Pathophysiologie der Analfissuren. Proktologie *1*, 55–58 (1980).

[221] ROSCHKE, W.: Die Entwicklungsmöglichkeiten der verschiedenen Hämorrhoidenformen, der Mariske, des Gleitanus und des Analprolapses. Colo-Proctology *1*, 33–39 (1981).

[222] ROSCHKE, W., KRAUSE, H.: Die proktologische Sprechstunde. Urban und Schwarzenberg, München (1986).

[223] ROUPAS, A., PACCAUD, M.F.: Les mycoplasures génitaux. Therapeutische Umschau 42, Heft *11*, 760–765 (1985).

[224] RUFLI, TH.: Sexuell übertragene Infektionskrankheiten des Anus und des Rektums. Schweiz. Rundschau Med. (Praxis) 72, Nr. *30*, 1000–1008 (1983).

[225] RUFLI, TH.: Die sexuell übertragenen Proktitiden des homosexuellen Mannes. Therapeutische Umschau 42, Heft *11*, 787–792 (1985).

[226] SAEUBERLI, H.: Colitis ulcerosa und Morbus Crohn – chirurgische Aspekte. Schweiz. Rundschau Med. (Praxis), *75*, 11, 283–289 (1986).

[227] SAINT-PIERRE, A., TREFFOT, M.J., MARTIN, P.M.: Hormone Receptors and Hemorrhoidal Disease. Colo-Proctology *2*, IV, 116–120 (1982).

[228] SAINT-PIERRE, A.: Problèmes posés par la présence de récepteurs hormonaux au niveau des hémorroïdes. Ann. Gastroenterol. Hépatol. *18*, 1, 19–27 (1982).

[229] SALMON, R.-J. et al.: Cancer du canal anal. Résultats du traitement d'une série de 195 cas. Gastroenterol. Clin. Biol. *9*, 911–917 (1985).

[230] SAMENIUS, B.: Perianal and Ano-rectal Condylomata Acuminata. Schweiz. Rundschau Med. (Praxis) 72, Nr. *30*, 1009–1014 (1983).

[231] SANDER, R.: Koloskopie-Brevier. F.K. Schattauer, Stuttgart (1982).

[232] SARLES, J.-C.: Symptomatologic et diagnostic différentiel des suppurations périanales et périnéales. Schweiz. Rundschau Med. (Praxis) 74, Nr. *35*, 905–908 (1985) + Encyclopédie méd. chir. Techniques chirurgicales. 40690 (1980).

[233] SARLES, J.-C.: Fissures anales et syndromes douloureux anaux. Revue du Praticien, 35, 3435–3441 (1985).

[234] SCHÄRLI, A.F., GEBBERS, J.-O.: Proktologische Probleme im Kindesalter. Hexagon «Roche» 13, Nr. *4*, Suppl. (1985).

[235] SCHÄRLI, A.F., GEBBERS, J.-O.: Proktologie im Kindesalter (Polyposissyndrome). Hexagon «Roche» 13, Nr. *6*, Suppl. (1985).

[236] SCHEURER, U.: Pseudomembranöse Kolitis. Schweiz. Rundschau Med. (Praxis) 73, Nr. *34*, 1027–1032 (1984).

[237] SCHMIDT, H., RIEMANN, J.F.: Melanosis coli und ihre klinische Bedeutung. Proktologie *1*, 11–15 (1980).

[238] SCHMITZ-MOORMANN, P., HIMMELMANN, W., BRANDES, H.-J.: Diagnostik anhand von Biopsiepräparaten. Z. Gastroenterologie *21*, 21–26 (1983).

[239] SCHNEIDER, K.W.: Anaphylaktischer Schock nach Sklerotherapie von Hämorrhoiden. Colo-Proctology *2*, 255–256 (1980).

[240] SCHNITZER, A.: Das Melanom, Ars Medici *2*, 58–63 (1986).

[241] SCHOUTEN, W.R., VAN VROONHOVEN, T.J.: Ambulante behandling von hemorrhoiden. Ned. Tijdschr. Geneeskd. *129* (21), 993–996 (1985).

[242] SCHUETZE, K., HENTSCHEL, E.: Klinik und Therapie der hämorrhagischen Proktitis. Wien. med. Wschr. *132*, 91–93 (1982).

[243] SCHUMANN, J., PETER, H.: Indikationen und Kontraindikationen der Analfisteloperation bei Morbus Crohn. Aktuelle Koloproktologie, Bd. 2, 42–43, Ed. Nymphenburg, München (1985).

[244] SCHWEIGER, M., ALEXANDER-WILLIAMS, J.: Das Ulkus simplex recti, seine Beziehung zum Rektumprolaps. Therapiewoche 29, 698–700 (1979).

[245] SEPULVEDA, B.: Progress in Amebiasis. Quadrennial Reviews, World Congress, Stockholm, Falkenberg, 153–164 (1982).

[246] SHPERBER, Y., HALEVY, A., BEN-ABARON, U.: Perianal tuberculosis, a case report. Isr. J. Med. Sci. 21 (5), 468–469 (1985).

[247] SMITH, L.E.: Symptomatic internal hemorrhoids. What are your options? Postgrad. Med. 73 (6), 323–330 (1983).

[248] SOULLARD, J.: Un procédé original de cryothérapie locale en proctologie le Zeroid. Gazette médicale de France, 80, 35, 5873–5880 (1973).

[249] SOULLARD, J., CONTOU, J.-F.: Colo-Proctologie. Masson, Paris (1984).

[250] SPIRO, P.: Hochdosierte lokale Heparintherapie in der Praxis. Schweiz. Rundschau Med. (Praxis) 69, Nr. 33, 1173–1177 (1980).

[251] STELZNER, F., STAUBESAND, J., MACHLEIDT, H.: Das Corpus cavernosum recti – die Grundlagen der innern Hämorrhoiden. Langenbecks Arch. Klin. Chir. 299, 302 (1962).

[252] STELZNER, F.: Die Hämorrhoiden und andere Krankheiten des Corpus cavernosum recti und des Analkanals. Dtsch. Med. Wochenschrift 88, 689 (1963).

[253] STELZNER, F.: Die anorektalen Fisteln. Springer Berlin, 2. Aufl. (1981).

[254] STEVEN, E. et al.: Herpes simplex virus proctitis in homosexuel men. New Engl. J. Med. 308, No. 15, 868–871 (1983).

[255] STEIN, E.: Praktische Erfahrungen mit der Sklerotherapie. Proktologie 2, 144–148 (1980).

[256] STEIN, E.: Das perianale Kontaktekzem. Colo-Proctology 5, 279–286 (1982).

[257] STEIN, E.: Proktologie, Lehrbuch und Atlas, Springer Verlag, Berlin (1986).

[258] STIRNEMANN, H.: Sakraldermoid und anale Plastikoperationen. Gastroent. Fortbildungsk. Praxis, Vol. 3, 54–59, Karger, Basel (1973).

[259] SULSER, H.: Pathologie der Kolonpolypen. Schweiz. Rundschau Med. (Praxis) 71, Nr. 27, 1127–1133 (1982).

[260] TEMPLETON, J.L., SPENCE, R.A.J., KENNEDY, T.L., PARKS, T.G., MACHENZIE, G., HANNA, W.A.: Comparison of infrered coagulation for first and second degree hemorrhoids: A randomised prospective clinical trial. Br. Med. J. I, 1387–1389 (1983).

[261] THEODORE, C., BAILLY, T., MOLAS, G., JULIEN, P.E., BARB, A., PAOLAGGI, J.A.: Colite à Salmonelle. Gastroenterol. Clin. Biol. 6, 943–944 (1982).

[262] THOMSON, H.: Die Pathologie der Hämorrhoiden. Colo-Proctology 1, 30–32 (1981).

[263] THOMSON, H.: The Nature of Piles. Schweiz. Rundschau Med. (Praxis) 71, 107–111 (1982).

[264] THOMSON, W.H.F.: The nature of the hemorrhoids. Arch. S. Surg. 62, 542 (1975).

[265] TRELLES, M.A., ROTINEN, S.: He/Ne laser treatment of hemorrhoids. Acupunct Electrother. Res. 8 (3–4), 289–295 (1983).

[266] TRIEHARNE, J.D.: Chlamydia trachomatis. Serological Diagnosis. Infection 10, Suppl. 1, 25 (1982).

[267] VANDENBROUCKE, J., VANTRAPPEN, G., TYTGAT, G., RUTGEERTS, L.: Morbus Crohn; in: Klinische Gastroenterologie, Vol. 1: Diagnostische Übersicht, Mundhöhle und Rachen, Speiseröhre, Magen, Darm, 386–398. Ed. L. Demling, Stuttgart: Thieme (1973).

[268] VANHEUVERZWYN, R. et al.: Chirurgisches Vorgehen beim analen Morbus Crohn. Colo-Proctology 2, 105–108 (1983).

[269] VANHEUVERZWYN, R.: Fistole anali. Piccin Ed. Padova (1979).

[270] VENDER, DJ., MARIGNANI, P.: Salmonella colitis presenting as a segmental colitis resembling Crohn's disease. Dis. Colon Rectum, 28, 848–851 (1983).

[271] VERNEUIL, A.: De l'hidrosadénite phlégmoneuse et des abcès sudoripares. Arch. Gen. Med. 114, 537–557 (1964).

[272] VIGNAL, J., RIVOIRE, M., DESCOS, L.: Les lésions ano-perianales de la Maladie de Crohn. Gastroentérologie Clinique et Biologique. 10, 2, 53A (1986).

[273] VOGT, M., LUETHY, R.: AIDS: Aktuelle Situation und heutiger Wissensstand. Therapeutische Umschau, Bd. 42, 798–804 (1985).

[274] WALSH, G., STICKLEY, G.S.: Acute Leukaemia with primary symptoms in the rectum. South med. J. 96, 684 (1934).

162

[275] WELIN, S., WELIN, C.: The Double Contrast Examination of the Colon. G. Thieme, Stuttgart (1976).

[276] WHITEHEAD, W.: Surgical treatment of hemorrhoids. Brit. med. J. *I,* 149 (1982).

[277] WILLIAMS, CH.B.: Koloskopie. In: Gastroenterologische Endoskopie, Ottenjann, R., Ferd. Enke Stuttgart, 183–197 (1979).

[278] WILLIAMS, K.L., HAG, I.H., ELEM, B.: Cryodestruction of Hemorrhoids. brit. med. J. *I,* 666 (1973).

[279] WINKLER, R.: Analfissur und Analfisteln. Therapiewoche *31,* 3779–3784 (1981).

[280] WITTEN, R.: Proktologie im alten Ägypten. Proktologie *2,* 18–20 (1979).

[281] WITZEL, L., HALTER, F., NEIGER, A.: Komplikationen der Fibersigmoidoskopie. In Fortschritte der gastroentereologischen Endoskopie. Witzstrock, Baden-Baden, 43–47 (1973).

[282] ZIMMER, S., PROBST, M., SCHROEDER, D.: Therapie des Basalioms der Anorektalregion. Fortschr. Med., 100. Jg., Nr. *13,* 571–574 (1982).

[283] ZIMMERLI, B., NEIGER, A., EGGER, G.: Die kurative endorektale Bestrahlung kleiner Rektum-Karzinome. Z. Gastroent. *83* (1971).

Subject Index